SIRTFOOD DIET COOKBOOK

•••

Get Lean, Feel Great, Burn fat with 500 Easy
and Tasty Recipes to Boost Your Metabolism

Simona Beck

What's Inside

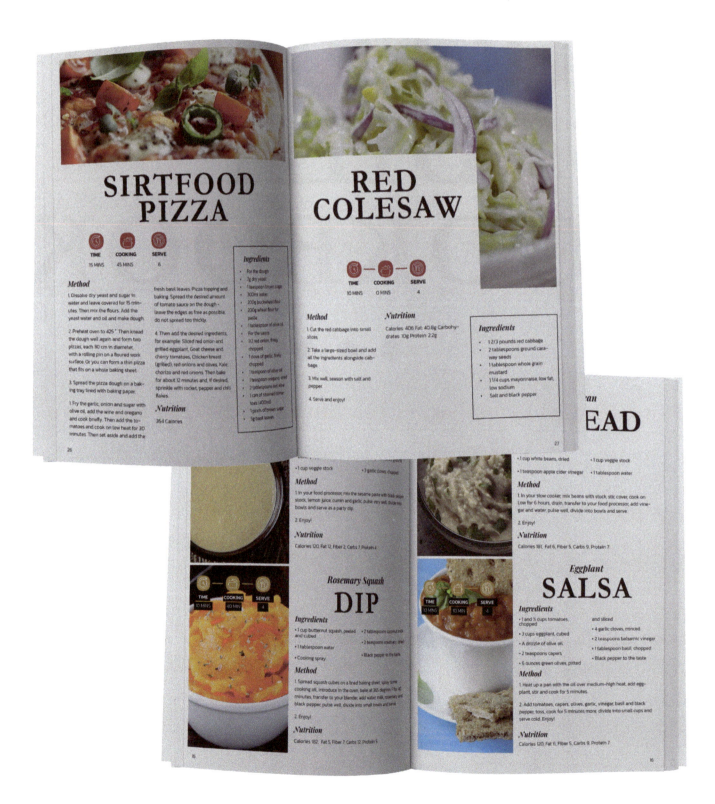

© Copyright 2020 All rights reserved.

Table Of Content

Chapter 1 — 06

Breakfast recipes - phase 1, Main meal recipes - phase 1, Dessert recipes - phase 1, Other recipes - phase 1, Breakfast recipes - phase 2, Main meal recipes - phase 2, Dessert recipes - phase 2, Other recipes - phase 1

Chapter 2 — 103

Fish: Savory Sirtfood Salmon, Fish With Mango and Turmeric, Sirtfood Shrimp Noodles, Sirtfood Miso Salmon, Sirtfood Salmon With Kale Salad, Sirtfood Shrimps With Buckwheat Noodles, Sirtfood Shellfish Salad

Chapter 3 — 111

Snacks: Sirtfood Pizza,

Chapter 4 — 115

Vegetarian Sirtfood Recipes: Breakfast, Lunch, Dinner

Chapter 5 — 130

Vegan Sirtfood Recipes: Breakfast, Lunch, Dinner

Chapter 6 — 145

Sirtfood Desserts: Sirtfood Walnut Balls, Sirtfood Brownies, Sirtfood Chocolate Mousse, Chocolate Sauce and Strawberry Pancakes, Cocoa and Medjool Dates Snacks, TWO-WEEK MEAL PLAN – PHASE 1 AND PHASE 2, Conclusion

Introduction

It would probably surprise you, but people knew about healthy foods long before we studied them in more recent years. In ancient times, they were discovering the effects of different plants and adopt some of them in their regular diet. Of course, back then, food was natural, so they weren't dealing with the same problem as we are dealing today. Thousands of years ago, people were dying for many causes; most of them were not related to bad nutrition. They didn't have the knowledge and technology to process food. Nowadays, medicine has evolved, but bad nutrition unfortunately causes plenty of deaths.

You are probably wondering how the Sirtfood diet was discovered. The founders of this meal plan have targeted the foods with a higher concentration of sirtuin-activating nutrients. They had a hunch about what these foods can do to your body. Then based on their findings, they have analyzed the eating habits and lifestyles of different people around the world who have a diet rich in sirtuin-activating nutrients. Therefore, if the Mediterranean diet was inspired by the eating habits and lifestyle of the people living on the Mediterranean shores, the Sirtfood diet tried the same approach, but this time, the analyzed population is spread all over the world.

There are regions from all over the world called the blue zones, where people eat plenty of sirtfoods. These people have a much lower rate of Alzheimer's disease, diabetes, heart disease, osteoporosis, and even cancer. Don't be surprised if you see people in their 90s walking, working, and dancing. This probably sounds like a fairy tale, a legend, or a myth, but there are people out there who are not affected by typical "western world" lifestyle. They don't have any stress, and they are enjoying life to the fullest.

If you have the privilege of visiting the San Blas Islands of Panama, you will definitely meet the Kuna American Indians, an indigenous population with incredibly low rates of high blood pressure, diabetes, obesity, cancer, and early deaths. Do you know what their secret is? It is the consumption of cocoa, which happens to have a high concentration of sirtuin-activating nutrients. Cocoa can increase memory performance and enhance brain functionality. It works miracles when it comes to preventing diabetes and even cancer, plus it can be used for better oral hygiene, as it can protect teeth from cavities and plaque.

Let's move on to India, which used to be the jewel in the crown of the British Empire. India can be easily considered a micro-continent, as its vast territory is home to some of the most amazing veggies, fruits, plants, and spices. Speaking of spices, do you know which spice is called the "Indian solid gold"? This is turmeric, and India is responsible for more than 80 percent of the global supply. This is a frequently used condiment in Indian cuisine and a great source of curcumin, a very powerful sirtuin-activating nutrient. As it turns out, the consumption of turmeric can have anti-inflammatory and healing effects. Curcumin has even anticancer effects, so it is better to have turmeric included in your diet.

China can be considered the home ground for green tea, one of the drinks with the most health benefits you can find out there. People in China have been drinking green tea for more than 4,700 years, and now this beverage has become extremely popular all over the world. The consumption of green tea can be associated with a lower risk of different forms of cancer (breast, prostate, breast, or lung) or lower rates of coronary heart disease. Green tea works wonders on metabolism, and it is the perfect drink to have when you want to burn fat while keeping your existing muscle mass intact.

If you have the pleasure of traveling in the Mediterranean region, you will notice how common the extra-virgin olive oil is for their daily diet. People living in this area like to consume healthy fats, and it looks like nuts (and especially walnuts) are a good source of lipids. Their diet is designed to burn fats in the body and keep the blood sugar and insulin level to a minimum, avoiding diabetes, obesity, heart diseases, and even some forms of cancer. No wonder there are so many people from this region who are aging slowly and feeling amazing.

If you take a look over the top 20 sirtfoods, you can easily see that some of the ingredients can only come from a specific region of the world. The Sirtfood diet practically brings the whole world on your plate so that you can reap the weight loss and health benefits of the best ingredients from all over the world.

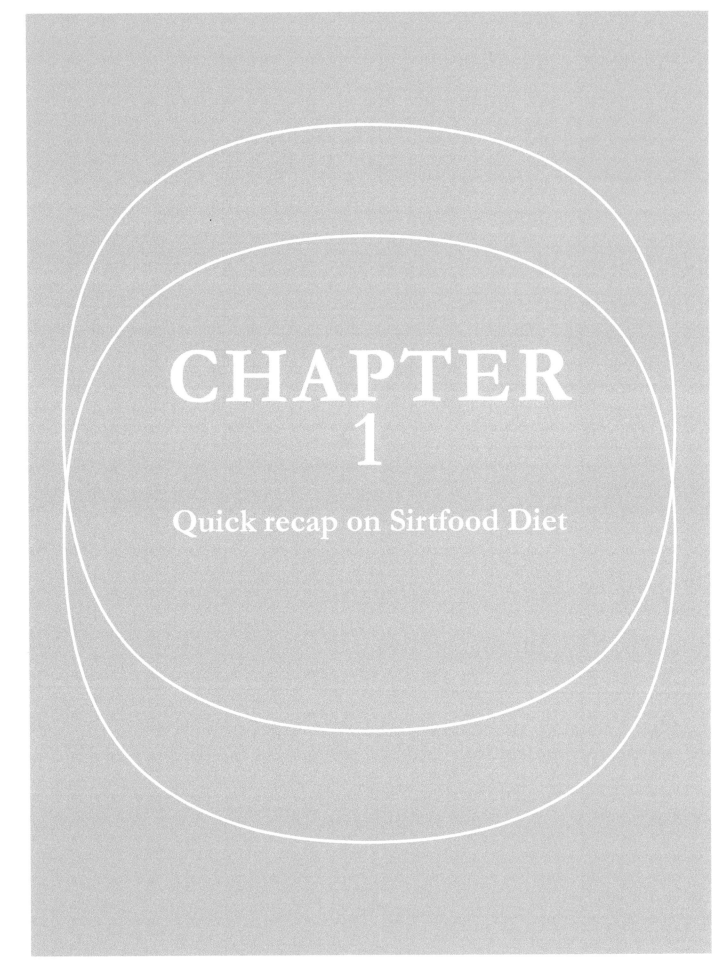

CHAPTER 1

Quick recap on Sirtfood Diet

Sirtfood Diet Phases

As a newbie, it is important you understand that the Sirtfood diet does not start with a single list of ingredients in your hands. Its implementation and adaptation are more than mere selective grocery shopping. Every diet can only work effectively when we allow our body to embrace the sudden shift and change in food intake. Similarly, the Sirtfood diet also comes with two phases of adaptation. Going through these phases, leads to following the Sirtfood diet easily and successfully. After the two weight loss phases, there is a third one which is basically a maintaining phase that aims to consolidate the weight loss results in the long run.

Phase One

The first seven days of this diet plan are known as Phase One. In this phase, a dieter must focus on calorie restriction and the intake of green juices. These seven days are crucial to initiate your weight loss and usually lead to lose up to seven pounds if the diet is followed properly. If you find yourself achieving this target that means that you are on the right track.

In the first three days of the Phase One, the caloric intake is set around to 1,000 calories. While doing so, the dieter must also have green juice throughout the day, three times per day. The recipes given in the book are perfect to select from. Pick a recipe given in their respective segments and pair each with green juices.

After the first three days and for the next four days, the caloric intake is increased to 1,500 calories per day. In these four days, the green juices to drink during the day are reduced to two, paired with Sirtuin-rich food in every meal.

Phase Two

Phase Two starts right after the first week of the Sirtfood diet or Phase One. It is about going on with the diet feeling it even easier thanks to body adaptation to the new regimen. The first week enables the body to embrace the change and start working towards the weight loss goal, according to the new diet. This phase enables the body to keep losing weight slowly and steadily. Therefore, the duration of this phase is almost two weeks.

So how is this phase different from the Phase One? In this phase, there is no restriction on the caloric intake, as long as the food is rich in sirtuins and you are having 3 meals per day. As far as green juices, the intake is decreased to one per day, which will be more than enough to guarantee weight loss. You can have the juice any time in the day, even after any meal, in the morning or in the evening.

After the Diet

With the end of Phase Two comes the time which is most crucial, and that is the after-diet phase. If you haven't achieved your weight loss target by the end of phase two, then you can restart the phases all over again. Or even when you have achieved the goals but still want to lose more weight.

Different Options for Every Need

The Sirtfood Diet, unlike fasting, doesn't involve skipping meals in order to experience the benefits it can offer. Therefore, you are not going through starvation to reach your weight loss and health goals. Nonetheless, the diet involves a very short period of caloric restriction that will require a bit of focus then you will increase calories again, going back to having breakfast, lunch, dinner, and snacks.
The Sirtfood Diet has been studied to meet the needs of the vast majority of people who need to lose weight.

Only people with serious illnesses, who are pregnant or breastfeeding should pay attention and skip to the maintenance phase, avoiding caloric restriction altogether. This means that they will still include healthy Sirtfoods (with their weight loss properties) in their everyday meals. They may not be able to take advantage of Phase 1 boost but still they will do the best choices for their health and weight loss.

Remember, even if you do not or cannot follow through with the restrictions, there is still a great benefit with adding the sirtuin-rich foods to your diet. As we will address shortly, many of the foods rich in sirtuins are highly nutritious and there is no doubt about the fact that they are very healthy and they should be included in your diet whether you want to follow the Sirtfood Diet or not.
Now you are probably wondering, "How am I going to lose pounds by eating three meals a day?"

The secret lies within the meal plan, as it can seriously deliver amazing results. Depending on the Phase you are in, you can enjoy eating dark chocolates and red wine while losing weight!
The average weight loss during the first week has been proved around seven pounds.
Of course not all bodies react the same to this diet, so the weight loss can be more or less visible but what this diet promises to deliver is that you will have outstanding results for trying it.

Once you are satisfied with the weight you reached, you can simply go into the maintenance phase of this diet and then transition to a normal healthy diet, still full of sirtuin-rich food. Sounds neat, right? This is what's great about this diet — it gives you the possibility to preserve your ideal weight long term, unlike many other radical diets where most people complain that they start to gain weight immediately after quitting.

The Sirtfood Diet Plan

The official Sirtfood Diet combines a short phase of calorie restriction with a long-term commitment to nutrient-dense sirtuin-activating foods. But before explaining how the diet is structured in detail, let's talk about two different and very important subjects when you are trying to achieve long lasting results.

The difference between Diet and Dieting

How you eat every day is your "diet", restricting how you eat is "dieting".
Aside from the first week, Phase 1, the Sirtfood diet is not a traditional diet in that: instead of simply restricting calories, you focus on increasing nutrition and improving quality of the food you eat.
There are two main phases in the Sirtfood Diet, which take up 3 weeks and are designed to set the stage for incorporating sirtfoods into your lifelong diet, eliminating your need to ever resort to dieting again and a third phase dedicated to transition to a normal (not restricted) healthy sirtfood-rich diet.
The average American over-consumes solid fats and sugars, refined grains, sodium, and saturated fat. They also under-consume vegetables, fruits, whole grains, as well as the nationally recommended intake of dairy and oils.
If this sounds like it matches your current eating patterns, don't be too hard on yourself, you're certainly not alone. And you've been practically brainwashed into adopting these poor nutrition habits.
The number of fast-food restaurants continues to grow, as do options for pre-made, packaged foods full of empty calories and misleading promises.
When you live on a diet of these foods that are lacking nutrition for too long, you find yourself getting sick and overweight.
How many times have you found yourself dieting, starving yourself for weeks to lose 20 pounds? Maybe you've even been successful a time or two and lost weight, but within a few months, all the weight you lost had found its way home again, and brought a few extra friends along.
Studies show that when you restrict your calories severely for an extended period of time, you will gain the weight back as quickly as it came off, and you will do additional damage to your liver, kidneys and muscle mass as well. Short term calorie restriction, such as the first phase of the Sirtfood Diet doesn't have the same effect as depleting your body of nutrition for a longer period.
To put it simply, dieting does not help you maintain the results you got in the long term.
More to the point, it's completely unnecessary. Think about many regions of the world, like Japan or the Mediterranean, where people traditionally don't count calories or diet, and they live to be 100+ with their full physical and mental capacities until one night, they drift off into a peaceful, joyous slumber never to wake again. That sounds a lot better than spending the last few months, if not years, of your life in a hospital bed, unable to wash or feed yourself, let alone walk around or remember your grandchildren.
You get to choose your future. And it begins with choosing a healthy diet rich in delicious, fortifying and age-defying sirtfoods.

Understanding Your Health Goals

You may have first heard about the Sirtfood Diet because you saw a headline about Adele's miraculous weight loss. Or perhaps you heard that scientists had discovered a "skinny gene" and the secret to accessing it was in this diet.

You want to lose weight, look great and feel great in your own skin.

That is a common and completely understandable desire, but it's not enough to get you the results you're dreaming of. At least not in the long-term. History has proven to us many times over that, even if we succeed in reaching our goal weight, either we're not satisfied or we are but we return to our old habits and the weight comes back.

One of the main reasons losing weight is ineffective is because it has an end or a result that you can achieve that allows you to give up.

If you start looking deeper and making a commitment to your health, you'll find that there is never a moment that you give yourself permission to stop. Even if you're relatively healthy today, you maintain a desire to stay healthy tomorrow, and following year, and 20 years from now. Health is a never-ending journey and that is where your true success and results will lie. You won't have a deadline to abide by and you can't fail, as long as you're taking actions every day that are designed to improve some aspect of your health.

Sometimes you'll see and feel the results right away. The participants in the first Sirtfood Diet trial saw weight loss results within 7 days. But other times, the benefits are on a cellular level and you won't realize they're making such a difference in your life until you're 80 years old and you the only one of your peers that hasn't been forced to move into assisted living.

One of the other major reasons dieting has a less than impressive track record is because of the type of weight loss that is occurring.

The diseases associated with obesity aren't caused only by excess weight. When you spend many years of eating unhealthy foods, you damage your metabolic system and the hormones that support your metabolism. Issues like insulin and leptin resistance cause you to gain weight and develop even more lethal diseases, like diabetes and heart disease. The food you eat is the problem, and the weight is simply a by-product of a dysfunctional metabolic system.

If you heal the system by removing the foods that are damaging your hormones and adding foods that will heal and protect your entire body, the weight will come off naturally as a result of fixing the damage.

When you try to take the weight off through calorie restriction, excessive exercise or a combination of the two, you will likely lower the numbers on your scale. There is truth to the philosophy of "calories in, calories out". However, if you aren't considering the quality of the calories going in, you won't have any control over what comes off. You're just as likely to lose water weight and muscle mass as you are to lose any fat.

If, on the other hand, you commit to providing your body with all the nutrition it needs to rebalance your hormones and protect your health, the weight that you lose is going to be the weight that you don't need: visceral fat around your vital organs and abdominal fat you've been struggling to get rid of for years. Your muscles will be protected and your body will stay nicely hydrated.

Losing weight as a result of improved health is sustainable, so it's crucial that you start to adjust your mindset and your goals if you truly want to be successful.

Not Only Weight Loss

Your weight is not the only thing you should be focusing on. Your health is the most important aspect of your life because, without it, you will have no joy and, most likely, very little hope of ever being able to maintain your ideal body weight.
If you prioritize health goals, you will have all the motivation you need to stop damaging your body with unhealthy foods with zero nutrition. You will be excited and inspired to try the myriad of fresh new ingredients that will help you feel lighter, younger, stronger and healthier than you can remember ever feeling.
The Sirtfood Diet is not about taking the easy route or popping a miracle cure pill. It's about finding the joy in your food and letting that food heal and nourish your body, allowing you to once again find joy in life. There are so many flavors waiting to be discovered, you simply need to commit to making sirtfoods the star players in your diet, with healthy proteins and fats as the phenomenal support team.
You don't have to starve yourself or even deny yourself the foods that you love, you simply have to approach food with mindfulness and awareness of the consequences it has on your body and your health.
The diet is mainly divided into two phases: the first lasts one week and the other lasts 14 days.

Phase 1 (The Most Effective): Three Kilos in Seven Days

It is the "supersonic" phase: the calorie restriction is combined with a diet rich in Sirt foods. The novelty compared to other diets is that it fattens and fattens the muscles. Two different moments. Days 1-3 are the most intense, and during this time you can consume a maximum of one thousand calories per day. You must consume 3 Sirt green juices and a solid meal.
On days 4-7 assigned the intake of one thousand five hundred calories daily. You have to take two green Sirt juices and two solid meals. Phase 1 is the most intense, in which the best results are seen and which allows you to lose up to 3.5 kilos.
The menu to follow includes a "fixed" part, the one relating to green juice created by nutritionists that helps to moderate the appetite of the brain, and one that varies daily.
The green juice recipe is simple and includes all-natural products: 75 g of curly kale, 30 g of arugula and 5 g of parsley must be centrifuged, together with 150 g of green celery with the leaves and 1/2 green apple, grated. Everything must be completed with half a squeezed lemon and half a teaspoon of Matcha tea.
Here is more in detail the program of the first week:
Monday – Wednesday: 3 Sirt green juices to be taken on waking up, mid-morning and mid-afternoon; 1 solid meal of animal or vegan protein (for example, turkey escalope or buckwheat noodles with tofu) accompanied by vegetables, always ending with 15-20 g of 85% dark chocolate.
Thursday – Sunday: 2 Sirt green juices and 2 solid meals, remembering to always vary the main course chosen, from salmon fillet to vegetable tabbouleh to buckwheat spaghetti with celery and kale.

Phase 2 (Maintenance), For 14 Days

Every day, for 14 days, you will eat three balanced meals, chock full of Sirt foods, drink a Sirt green juice and consume 1-2 Sirt snacks. Green juice should be taken in the morning as soon as you wake up or at least 30 minutes before breakfast, or mid-morning. The evening meal must be eaten by 7pm.

Phase 2 is the maintenance phase. During this period the goal is the consolidation of weight loss, although the possibility of losing weight is not excluded. To do all this, just feed on the exceptional food's rich in sirtuins. It lasts 14 days, is less restrictive than the first and provides for sirt foods at will: 3 solid meals plus two juices. The important thing is that they are balanced.

The positive aspects of this diet are :

One is the fact that the calorie limit is indicative and not a goal to be achieved. Another advantage is that the dishes on offer are very satisfying. This way you won't have the hunger attacks typical of other diets. The caloric restriction of the diet even in the most intensive phase is not drastic and Sirt foods have a satiating effect, which prevents us from getting hungry at meals.

And then?

As already explained in the introduction, the sirtfood diet cannot (and must not) continue indefinitely and for a very long period of time. Rather, it must be done in cycles, once, two or three times a year. However, the "lifestyle" sirt can continue even after completing the phase. Sirt foods can be eaten all year round, continuing to speed up the metabolism. However, this should not be combined with a very strong calorie restriction, but only avoid eating unhealthy foods, such as fried, sweet or unsaturated fats. Your persistence will make the difference between success and failure, remember: this is not a shot, but a marathon!

Sirt cycles are simply a boost, a powerful weapon in your arsenal that you can use twice a year (depending on your body of course), but you can have a healthy lifestyle all year round, perhaps combined with a regular physical exercise.

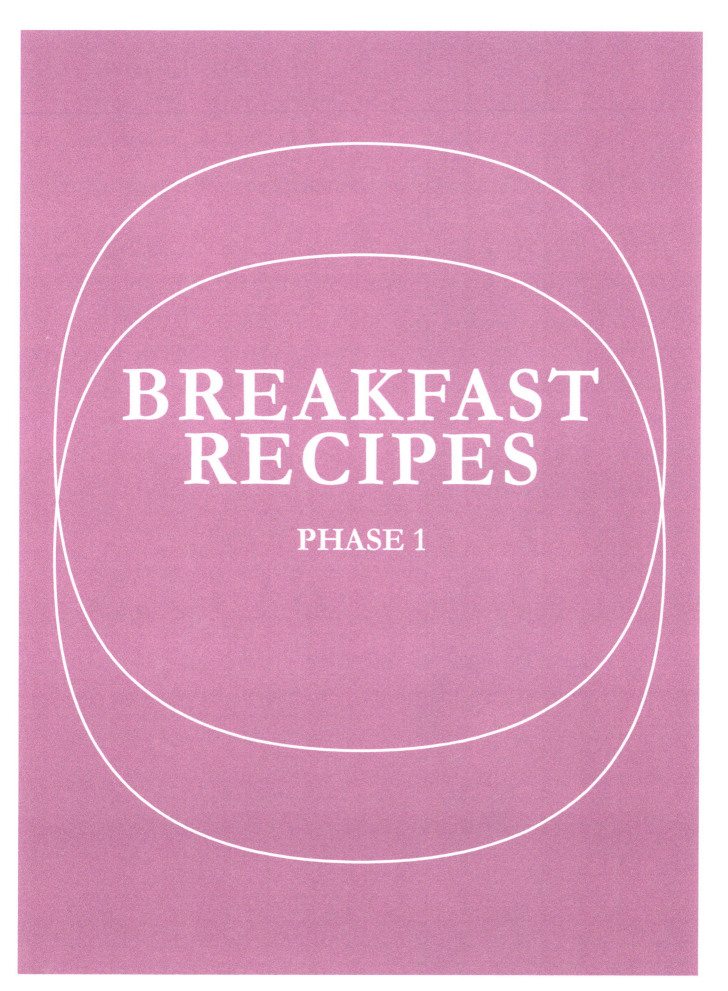

Main Baby Spinach SNACK

Ingredients

- 2 cups baby spinach, washed
- A pinch of black pepper
- ½ tablespoon olive oil
- ½ teaspoon garlic powder

Method

1. Spread the baby spinach on a lined baking sheet, add oil, black pepper and garlic powder, toss a bit, introduce in the oven, bake at 350 degrees F for 10 minutes, divide into bowls and serve as a snack.

2. Enjoy!

Nutrition

Calories 125, Fat 4, Fiber 1, Carbs, 4 Protein 2

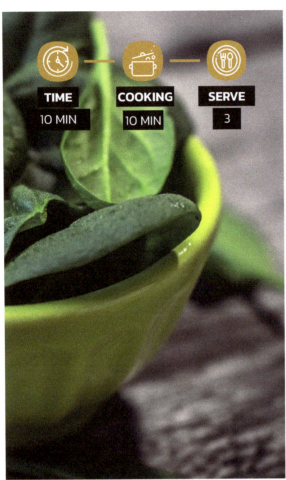

Potato BITES

Ingredients

- 1 potato, sliced
- 2 bacon slices, already cooked and crumbled
- 1 small avocado, pitted and cubed
- Cooking spray

Method

1. Spread potato slices on a lined baking sheet, spray with cooking oil, introduce in the oven at 350 degrees F, bake for 20 minutes, arrange on a platter, top each slice with avocado and crumbled bacon and serve as a snack.

2. Enjoy!

Nutrition

Calories 180, Fat 4, Fiber 1, Carbs 8, Protein 6

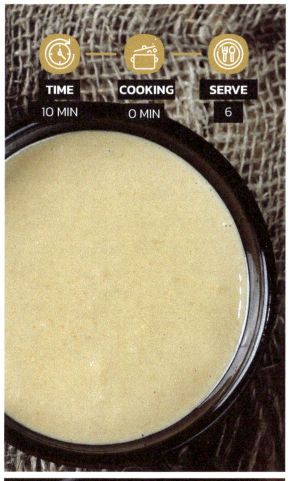

Sesame DIP

TIME 10 MIN | **COOKING** 0 MIN | **SERVE** 6

Ingredients

- 1 cup sesame seed paste, pure
- Black pepper to the taste
- 1 cup veggie stock
- ½ cup lemon juice
- ½ teaspoon cumin, ground
- 3 garlic cloves, chopped

Method

1. In your food processor, mix the sesame paste with black pepper, stock, lemon juice, cumin and garlic, pulse very well, divide into bowls and serve as a party dip.

2. Enjoy!

Nutrition

Calories 120, Fat 12, Fiber 2, Carbs 7, Protein 4

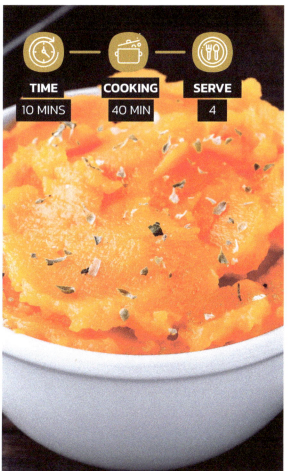

Rosemary Squash DIP

TIME 10 MINS | **COOKING** 40 MIN | **SERVE** 4

Ingredients

- 1 cup butternut squash, peeled and cubed
- 1 tablespoon water
- Cooking spray
- 2 tablespoons coconut milk
- 2 teaspoons rosemary, dried
- Black pepper to the taste

Method

1. Spread squash cubes on a lined baking sheet, spray some cooking oil, introduce in the oven, bake at 365 degrees F for 40 minutes, transfer to your blender, add water, milk, rosemary and black pepper, pulse well, divide into small bowls and serve

2. Enjoy!

Nutrition

Calories 182, Fat 5, Fiber 7, Carbs 12, Protein 5

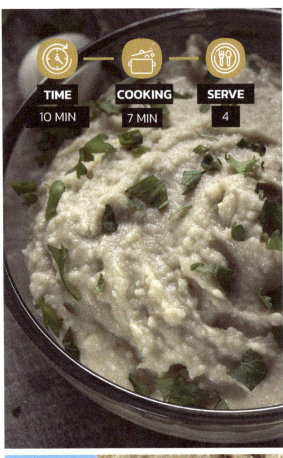

Bean
SPREAD

Ingredients

- 1 cup white beans, dried
- 1 teaspoon apple cider vinegar
- 1 cup veggie stock
- 1 tablespoon water

Method

1. In your slow cooker, mix beans with stock, stir, cover, cook on Low for 6 hours, drain, transfer to your food processor, add vinegar and water, pulse well, divide into bowls and serve.

2. Enjoy!

Nutrition

Calories 181, Fat 6, Fiber 5, Carbs 9, Protein 7

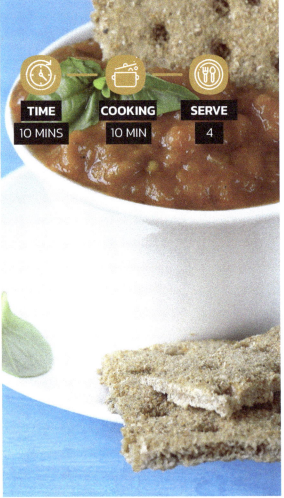

Eggplant
SALSA

Ingredients

- 1 and ½ cups tomatoes, chopped
- 3 cups eggplant, cubed
- A drizzle of olive oil
- 2 teaspoons capers
- 6 ounces green olives, pitted and sliced
- 4 garlic cloves, minced
- 2 teaspoons balsamic vinegar
- 1 tablespoon basil, chopped
- Black pepper to the taste

Method

1. Heat up a pan with the oil over medium-high heat, add eggplant, stir and cook for 5 minutes.

2. Add tomatoes, capers, olives, garlic, vinegar, basil and black pepper, toss, cook for 5 minutes more, divide into small cups and serve cold. Enjoy!

Nutrition

Calories 120, Fat 6, Fiber 5, Carbs 9, Protein 7

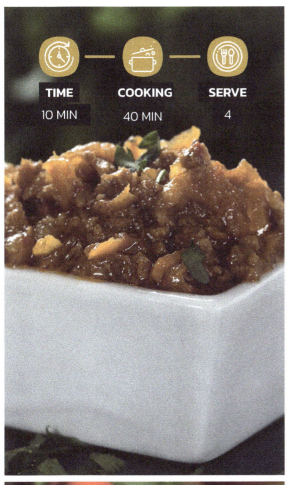

Carrots and Cauliflower SPREAD

TIME 10 MIN | **COOKING** 40 MIN | **SERVE** 4

Ingredients

- 1 cup carrots, sliced
- 2 cups cauliflower florets
- ½ cup cashews
- 2 and ½ cups water
- 1 cup almond milk
- 1 teaspoon garlic powder
- ¼ teaspoon smoked paprika

Method

1. In a small pot, mix the carrots with cauliflower, cashews and water, stir, cover, bring to a boil over medium heat, cook for 40 minutes, drain and transfer to a blender.

2. Add almond milk, garlic powder and paprika, pulse well, divide into small bowls and serve. Enjoy!

Nutrition

Calories 201, Fat 7, Fiber 4, Carbs 7, Protein 7

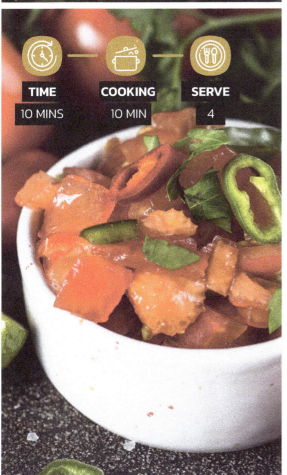

Italian Veggie SALSA

TIME 10 MINS | **COOKING** 10 MIN | **SERVE** 4

Ingredients

- 2 red bell peppers, cut into medium wedges
- 3 zucchinis, sliced
- ½ cup garlic, minced
- 2 tablespoons olive oil
- A pinch of black pepper
- 1 teaspoon Italian seasoning

Method

1. Heat up a pan with the oil over medium-high heat, add bell peppers and zucchini, toss and cook for 5 minutes.

2. Add garlic, black pepper and Italian seasoning, toss, cook for 5 minutes more, divide into small cups and serve as a snack.

3. Enjoy!

Nutrition

Calories 132, Fat 3, Fiber 3, Carbs 7, Protein 4

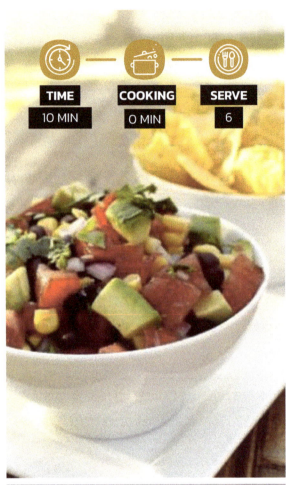

Black Bean SALSA

Ingredients

- 1 tablespoon coconut aminos
- ½ teaspoon cumin, ground
- 1 cup canned black beans, no-salt-added, drained and rinsed
- 1 cup salsa
- 6 cups romaine lettuce leaves, torn
- ½ cup avocado, peeled, pitted and cubed

Method

1. In a bowl, combine the beans with the aminos, cumin, salsa, lettuce and avocado, toss, divide into small bowls and serve as a snack.

2. Enjoy!

Nutrition

Calories 181, Fat 4, Fiber 7, Carbs 14, Protein 7

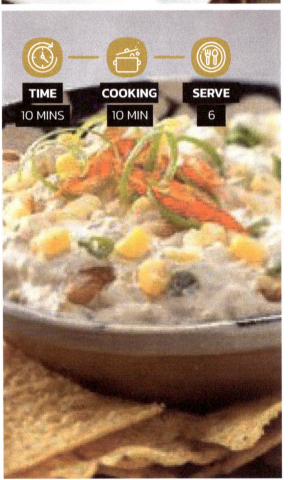

Corn SPREAD

Ingredients

- 30 ounces canned corn, drained
- 2 green onions, chopped
- ½ cup coconut cream
- 1 jalapeno, chopped
- ½ teaspoon chili powder

Method

1. In a small pan, combine the corn with green onions, jalapeno and chili powder, stir, bring to a simmer, cook over medium heat for 10 minutes, leave aside to cool down, add coconut cream, stir well, divide into small bowls and serve as a spread.

2. Enjoy!

Nutrition

Calories 192, Fat 5, Fiber 10, Carbs 11, Protein 8

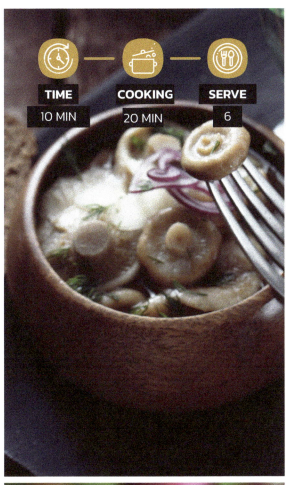

Mushroom DIP

TIME 10 MIN — **COOKING** 20 MIN — **SERVE** 6

Ingredients

- 1 cup yellow onion, chopped
- 3 garlic cloves, minced
- 1-pound mushrooms, chopped
- 28 ounces tomato sauce, no-salt-added
- Black pepper to the taste

Method

1. Put the onion in a pot, add garlic, mushrooms, black pepper and tomato sauce, stir, cook over medium heat for 20 minutes, leave aside to cool down, divide into small bowls and serve.

2. Enjoy!

Nutrition

Calories 215, Fat 4, Fiber 7, Carbs 3, Protein 7

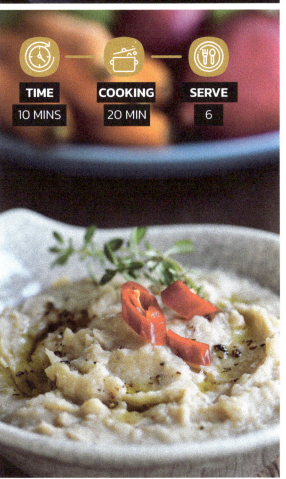

Salsa Bean DIP

TIME 10 MINS — **COOKING** 20 MIN — **SERVE** 6

Ingredients

- ½ cup salsa
- 2 cups canned white beans, no-salt-added, drained and rinsed
- 1 cup low-fat cheddar, shredded
- 2 tablespoons green onions, chopped

Method

1. In a small pot, combine the beans with the green onions and salsa, stir, bring to a simmer over medium heat, cook for 20 minutes, add cheese, stir until it melts, take off heat, leave aside to cool down, divide into bowls and serve.

2. Enjoy!

Nutrition

Calories 212, Fat 5, Fiber 6, Carbs 10, Protein 8

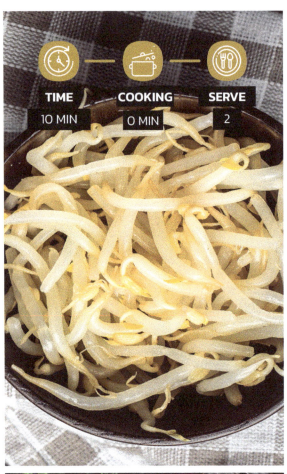

Mung Sprouts SALSA

Ingredients

- 1 red onion, chopped
- 2 cups mung beans, sprouted
- A pinch of red chili powder
- 1 green chili pepper, chopped
- 1 tomato, chopped
- 1 teaspoon chaat masala
- 1 teaspoon lemon juice
- 1 tablespoon coriander, chopped
- Black pepper to the taste

Method

1. In a salad bowl, mix onion with mung sprouts, chili pepper, tomato, chili powder, chaat masala, lemon juice, coriander and pepper, toss well, divide into small cups and serve.

2. Enjoy!

Nutrition

Calories 100, Fat 2, Fiber 1, Carbs 3, Protein 6

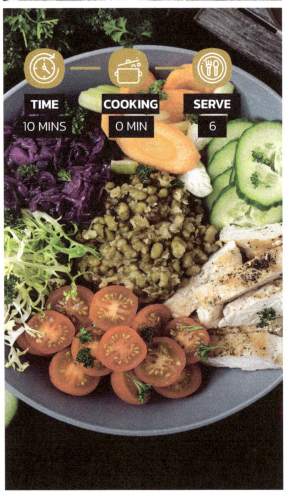

Mung Beans Snack SALAD

Ingredients

- 2 cups tomatoes, chopped
- 2 cups cucumber, chopped
- 3 cups mixed greens
- 2 cups mung beans, sprouted
- 2 cups clover sprouts
- For the salad dressing:
- 1 tablespoon cumin, ground
- 1 cup dill, chopped
- 4 tablespoons lemon juice
- 1 avocado, pitted, peeled and roughly chopped
- 1 cucumber, roughly chopped

Method

1. In a salad bowl, mix tomatoes with 2 cups cucumber, greens, clover and mung sprouts.

2. In your blender, mix cumin with dill, lemon juice, 1 cucumber and avocado, blend really well, add this to your salad, toss well and serve as a snack. Enjoy!

Nutrition

Calories 120, Fat 0, Fiber 2, Carbs 1, Protein 6

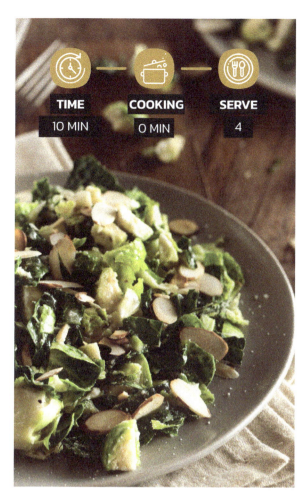

TIME 10 MIN | **COOKING** 0 MIN | **SERVE** 4

Sprouts and Apples Snack
SALAD

Ingredients

- 1-pound Brussels sprouts, shredded
- 1 cup walnuts, chopped
- 1 apple, cored and cubed
- 1 red onion, chopped
- For the salad dressing:
- 3 tablespoons red vinegar
- 1 tablespoon mustard
- ½ cup olive oil
- 1 garlic clove, minced
- Black pepper to the taste

Method

1. In a salad bowl, mix sprouts with apple, onion and walnuts.

2. In another bowl, mix vinegar with mustard, oil, garlic and pepper, whisk really well, add this to your salad, toss well and serve as a snack. Enjoy!

Nutrition

Calories 125, Fat 4, Fiber 1, Carbs, 4 Protein 2

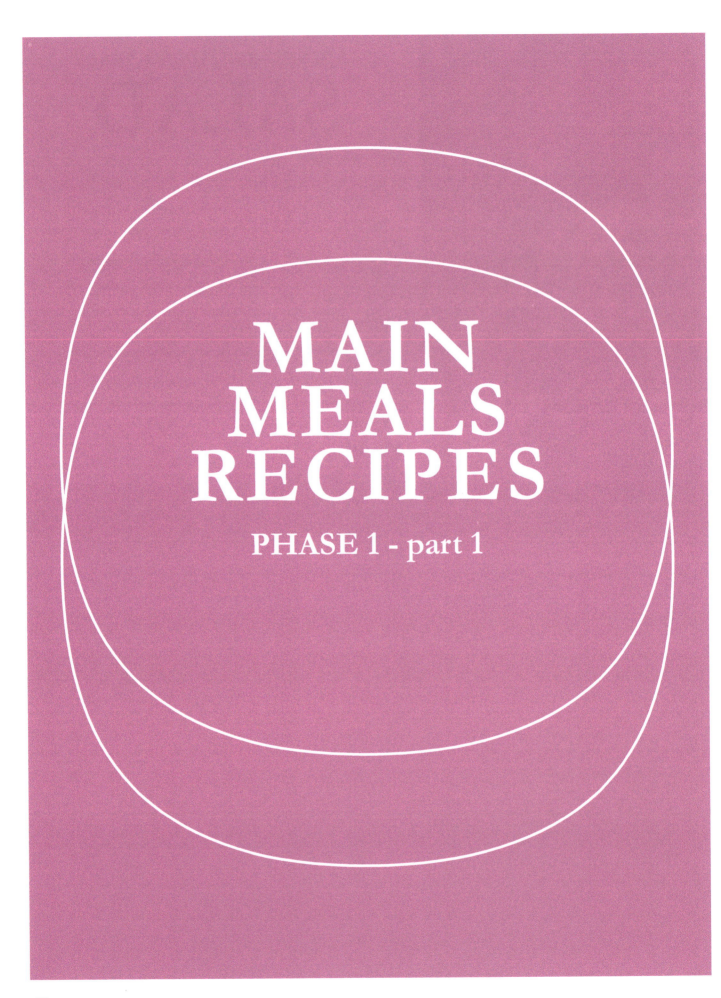
MAIN MEALS RECIPES

PHASE 1 - part 1

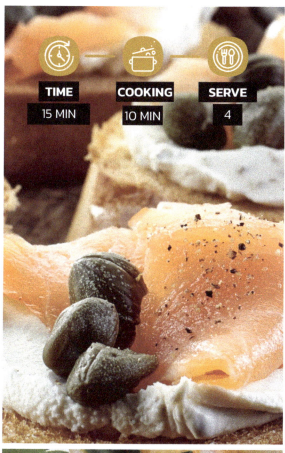

Salmon and CAPERS

TIME 15 MIN | **COOKING** 10 MIN | **SERVE** 4

Ingredients

- 75g (3oz) Greek yogurt
- 4 salmon fillets, skin removed
- 4 teaspoons Dijon Mustard
- 1 tablespoon capers, chopped
- 2 teaspoons fresh parsley
- Zest of 1 lemon

Method

1. In a bowl, mix together the yogurt, mustard, lemon zest, parsley and capers. Thoroughly coat the salmon in the mixture. Place the salmon under a hot grill (broiler) and cook for 3-4 minutes on each side, or until the fish is cooked. Serve with mashed potatoes and vegetables or a large green leafy salad.

Nutrition

321 calories per serving.

Coconut CURRY

TIME 10 MINS | **COOKING** 2 MIN | **SERVE** 4

Ingredients

- 400g (14oz) tinned chopped tomatoes
- 25g (1oz) fresh coriander (cilantro) chopped
- 3 red onions, finely chopped
- 3 cloves of garlic, crushed
- 2 bird's eye chillies
- ½ teaspoon ground coriander (cilantro)
- ½ teaspoon turmeric
- 400mls (14fl oz.) coconut milk
- 1 tablespoons olive oil
- Juice of 1 lime

Method

1. Place the onions, garlic, tomatoes, chillies, lime juice, turmeric, ground coriander (cilantro), chillies and half of the fresh coriander (cilantro) into a blender and blitz until you have a smooth curry paste. Heat the olive oil in a frying pan, add the paste and cook for 2 minutes. Stir in the coconut milk and warm it thoroughly. Stir in the fresh coriander (cilantro). Serve with rice

Nutrition

322 calories per serving.

Turkey CURRY

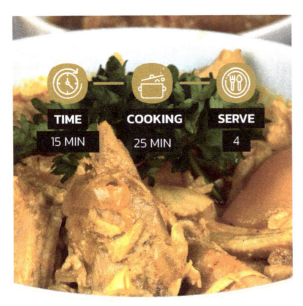

TIME 15 MIN
COOKING 25 MIN
SERVE 4

Ingredients

- 450g (1lb) turkey breasts, chopped
- 100g (3½ oz.) fresh rocket (arugula) leaves, 5 cloves garlic, chopped
- 3 teaspoons medium curry powder
- 2 teaspoons turmeric powder
- 2 tablespoons fresh coriander (cilantro), finely chopped
- 2 bird's-eye chillies, chopped
- 2 red onions, chopped
- 400mls (14fl oz.) full-fat coconut milk
- 2 tablespoons olive oil

Method

1. Heat the olive oil in a saucepan, add the chopped red onions and cook them for around 5 minutes or until soft. Stir in the garlic and the turkey and cook it for 7-8 minutes. Stir in the turmeric, chillies and curry powder then add the coconut milk and coriander (cilantro). Bring it to the boil, reduce the heat and simmer for around 10 minutes. Scatter the rocket (arugula) onto plates and spoon the curry on top. Serve alongside brown rice.

Nutrition

402 calories per serving.

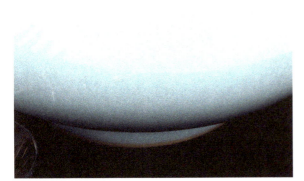

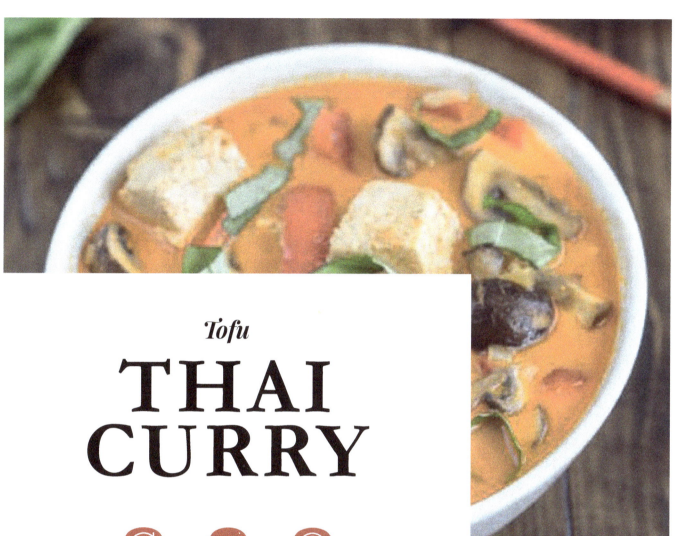

Tofu THAI CURRY

TIME	COOKING	SERVE
15 MINS	15 MINS	4

Method

1. Heat the oil in a frying pan, add the onion and cook for 4 minutes. Add in the chillies, cumin, ginger, and garlic and cook for 2 minutes. Add the tomato puree, lemon grass, sugar-snap peas, lime juice and tofu and cook for 2 minutes. Pour in the stock (broth), coconut milk and coriander (cilantro) and simmer for 5 minutes. Serve with brown rice or buckwheat and a handful of rockets (arugula) leaves on the side.

Nutrition

270 calories per serving.

Ingredients

- 400g (14oz) tofu, diced
- 200g (7oz) sugar snap peas
- 5cm (2 inch) chunk fresh ginger root, peeled and finely chopped
- 2 red onions, chopped, 2 cloves of garlic, crushed
- 2 bird's eye chillies
- 2 tablespoons tomato puree
- 1 stalk of lemon grass, inner stalks only
- 1 tablespoon fresh coriander (cilantro), chopped
- 1 teaspoon cumin
- 300mls (½ pint) coconut milk
- 200mls (7fl oz.) vegetable stock (broth)
- 1 tablespoon virgin olive oil
- Juice of 1 lime

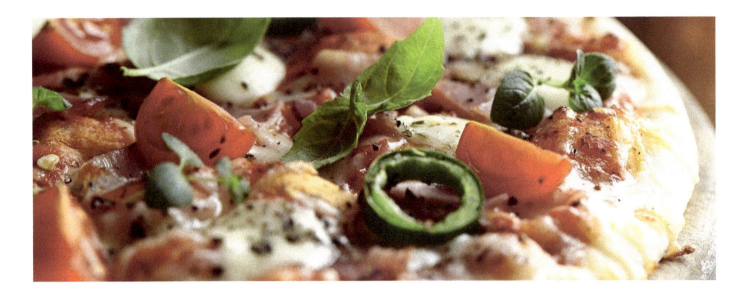

SIRTFOOD PIZZA

TIME
15 MINS

COOKING
45 MINS

SERVE
6

Method

1. Dissolve dry yeast and sugar in water and leave covered for 15 minutes. Then mix the flours. Add the yeast water and oil and make dough.

2. Preheat oven to 425 °. Then knead the dough well again and form two pizzas, each 30 cm in diameter, with a rolling pin on a floured work surface. Or you can form a thin pizza that fits on a whole baking sheet.

3. Spread the pizza dough on a baking tray lined with baking paper.

1. Fry the garlic, onion and sugar with olive oil, add the wine and oregano and cook briefly. Then add the tomatoes and cook on low heat for 30 minutes. Then set aside and add the fresh basil leaves. Pizza topping and baking. Spread the desired amount of tomato sauce on the dough - leave the edges as free as possible, do not spread too thickly.

4. Then add the desired ingredients, for example: Sliced red onion and grilled eggplant, Goat cheese and cherry tomatoes, Chicken breast (grilled), red onions and olives, Kale, chorizo and red onions. Then bake for about 12 minutes and, if desired, sprinkle with rocket, pepper and chili flakes.

Nutrition

354 Calories.

Ingredients

- For the dough
- 7g dry yeast
- 1 teaspoon brown sugar
- 300ml water
- 200g buckwheat flour
- 200g wheat flour for pasta
- 1 tablespoon of olive oil
- For the sauce
- 1/2 red onion, finely chopped
- 1 clove of garlic, finely chopped
- 1 teaspoon of olive oil
- 1 teaspoon oregano, dried
- 2 tablespoons red wine
- 1 can of strained tomatoes (400ml)
- 1 pinch of brown sugar
- 5g basil leaves

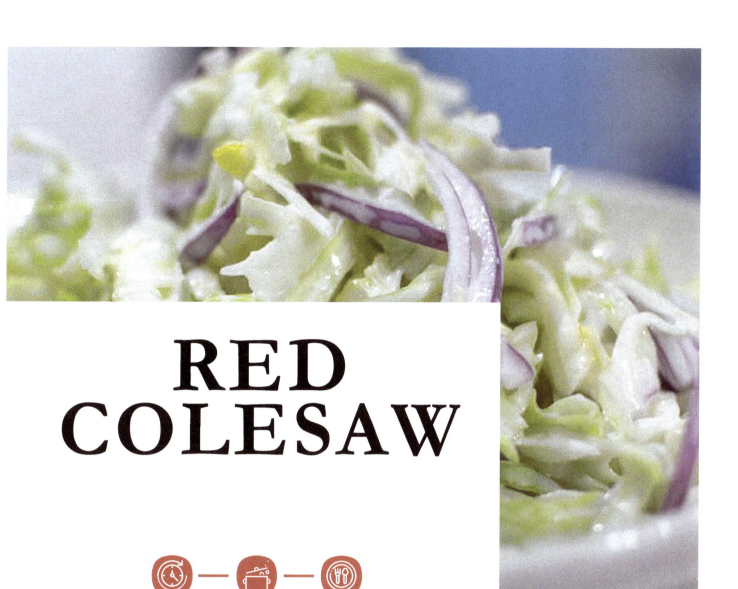

RED COLESAW

TIME 10 MINS — **COOKING** 0 MINS — **SERVE** 4

Method

1. Cut the red cabbage into small slices.

2. Take a large-sized bowl and add all the ingredients alongside cabbage.

3. Mix well, season with salt and pepper.

4. Serve and enjoy!

Nutrition

Calories: 406 Fat: 40.8g Carbohydrates: 10g Protein: 2.2g

Ingredients

- 1 2/3 pounds red cabbage
- 2 tablespoons ground caraway seeds
- 1 tablespoon whole grain mustard
- 1 1/4 cups mayonnaise, low fat, low sodium
- Salt and black pepper

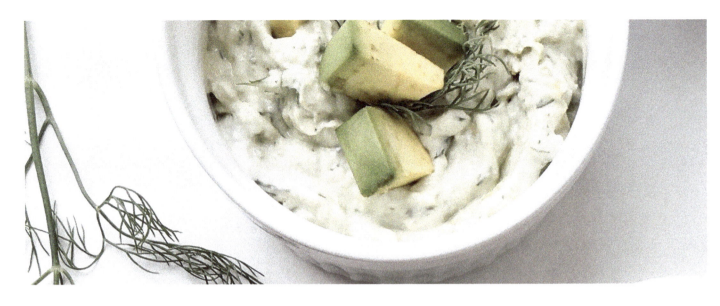

Avocado Mayo
MEDLEY

TIME   **COOKING**   **SERVE**

5 MINS   0 MINS   4

Method

1. Take a food processor and add avocado, cayenne pepper, lime juice, salt and cilantro.

2. Mix until smooth.

3. Slowly incorporate olive oil, add 1 tablespoon at a time and keep processing between additions.

4. Store and use as needed!

Nutrition

Calories: 231 Fat: 20g Carbohydrates: 5g Protein: 3g

Ingredients

- 1 medium avocado, cut into chunks
- ½ teaspoon ground cayenne pepper
- 2 tablespoons fresh cilantro
- ¼ cup olive oil
- ½ cup mayo, low fat and los sodium

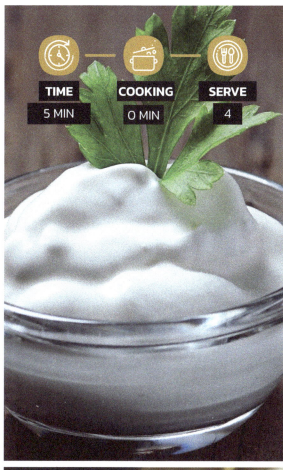

Amazing Garlic
AIOLI

TIME 5 MIN · **COOKING** 0 MIN · **SERVE** 4

Ingredients

- ½ cup mayonnaise, low fat and low sodium
- 2 garlic cloves, minced
- Juice of 1 lemon
- 1 tablespoon fresh-flat leaf Italian parsley, chopped
- 1 teaspoon chives, chopped
- Salt and pepper to taste

Method

2. Add mayonnaise, garlic, parsley, lemon juice, chives and season with salt and pepper.

3. Blend until combined well.

4. Pour into refrigerator and chill for 30 minutes.

5. Serve and use as needed!

Nutrition

Calories: 813 Fat: 88g Carbohydrates: 9g Protein: 2g

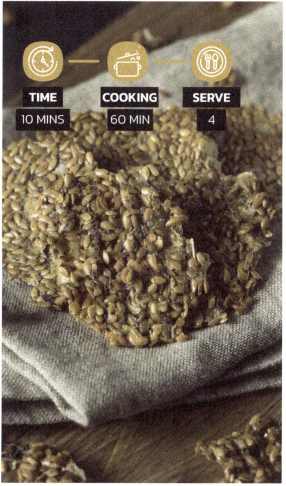

Easy Seed
CREACKERS

TIME 10 MINS · **COOKING** 60 MIN · **SERVE** 4

Ingredients

- 1 cup boiling water
- 1/3 cup chia seeds
- 1/3 cup sesame seeds
- 1/3 cup pumpkin seeds
- 1/3 cup Flaxseeds
- 1/3 cup sunflower seeds
- 1 tablespoon Psyllium powder
- 1 cup almond flour
- 1 teaspoon salt
- ¼ cup coconut oil, melted

Method

Pre-heat your oven to 300 degrees F. Line a cookie sheet with parchment paper and keep it on the side. Add listed ingredients (except coconut oil and water) to food processor and pulse until ground. Transfer to a large mixing bowl and pour melted coconut oil and boiling water, mix. Transfer mix to prepared sheet and spread into a thin layer. Cut dough into crackers and bake for 60 minutes. Cool and serve. Enjoy!

Nutrition

Total Carbs: 10.6g Fiber: 3g Protein: 5g Fat: 14.6g

MAIN MEALS RECIPES

PHASE 1 - part 2

Sticky Chicken Watermelon

NOODLE SALAD

TIME   **COOKING**   **SERVE**

10 MINS   6 MINS   3

Method

1. In a bowl, then completely substituting the noodles in boiling drinking water. They are going to soon be spread out in 2 minutes.

2. On a big sheet of parchment paper, throw the chicken with pepper, salt and also the five-spice.

3. Twist over the paper, subsequently flatten the chicken using a rolling pin. Place into the large skillet with 1 tbsp. of olive oil, turning 3 or 4 minutes, until well charred and cooked through.

5. Drain the noodles and toss with 1 tbsp. of sesame oil onto a sizable serving dish. Place 50% the noodles into the moderate skillet, stirring frequently until crispy and nice.

7. Remove the watermelon skin, then slice the flesh to inconsistent balls and then move to plate.

8. Wash the lettuces and cut into small wedges and also half of a whole lot of leafy greens and scatter on the dish. Place another 1 / 2 the cilantro pack, the soy sauce, coriander, chives, peanut butter, a dab of water, 1 teaspoon of sesame oil and the lime juice in a bowl, then mix till smooth.

10. Set the chicken back to heat, garnish with all the sweet sauce (or my walnut syrup mixture) and toss with the sesame seeds.

11. Pour the dressing on the salad toss gently with clean fingers until well coated, then add crispy noodles and then smashed cashews.

12. Mix chicken pieces and add them to the salad.

Nutrition

254 calories

Ingredients

- 2 pieces of skinny rice noodles
- 1/2 tbsp. sesame oil, 2 cups watermelon
- Head of bib lettuce, Half of a lot of scallions
- Half of a lot of fresh cilantro
- 2 skinless, boneless chicken breasts
- 1/2 tbsp. Chinese five-spice, 1 tbsp. extra virgin olive oil
- Two tbsp. sweet skillet (I utilized a mixture of maple syrup using a dash of tabasco)
- 1 tbsp. sesame seeds, A couple of cashews - smashed
- Dressing - could be made daily or 2 until
- 1 tbsp. low-salt soy sauce
- 1 teaspoon sesame oil, 1 tbsp. peanut butter
- Half of a refreshing red chili
- Half of a couple of chives
- Half of a couple of cilantros
- 1 lime - juiced
- 1 small spoonful of garlic

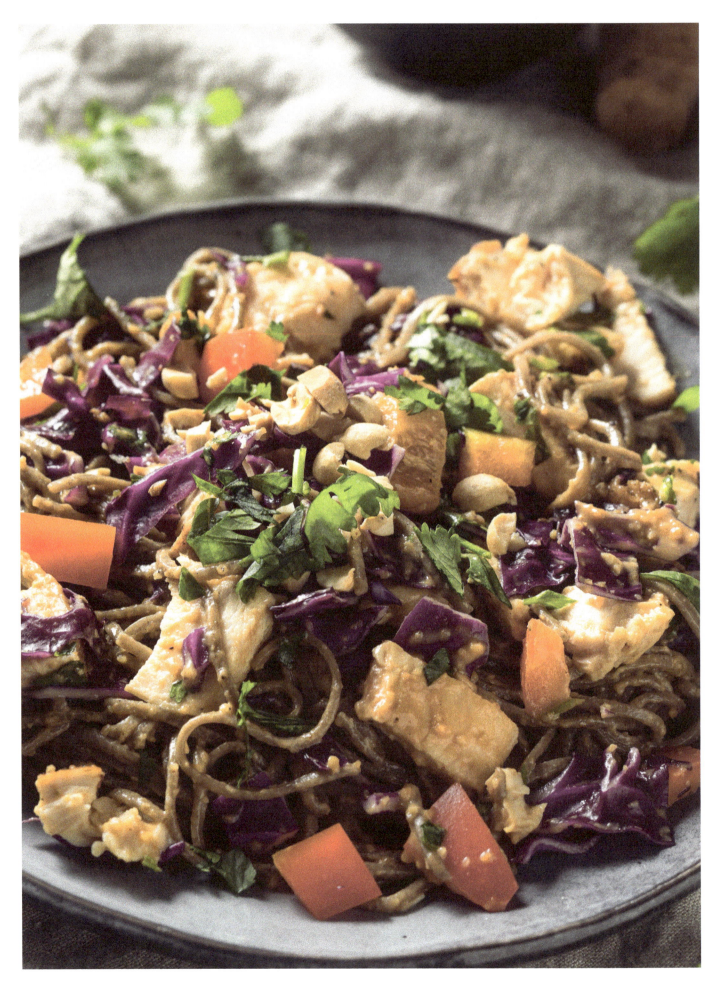

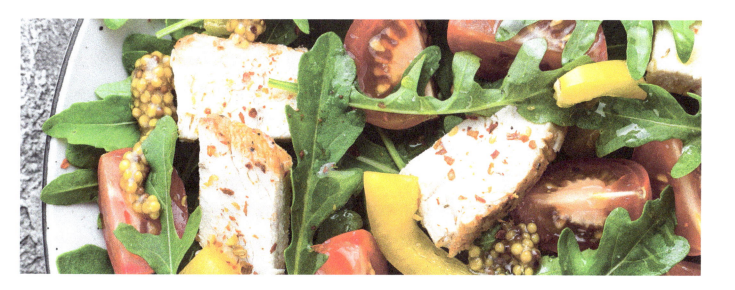

Fruity Curry

CHICKEN SALAD

TIME   **COOKING**   **SERVE**

15 MINS   0 MINS   2

Method

1. In a big bowl combine the chicken, onion, celery, apple, celery, celery, pecans, pepper, curry powder, and carrot. Mix altogether.

2. Enjoy!

Nutrition

Per serving: 229 carbohydrates 14 grams total fat 44 milligrams cholesterol

Ingredients

- 4 skinless, boneless chicken pliers – cooked and diced
- 1 tsp. celery, diced
- 4 green onions, sliced
- 1 golden delicious apple peeled, cored and diced
- 1/3 cup golden raisins
- 1/3 cup seedless green grapes, halved
- 1/2 cup sliced toasted pecans
- ⅛ Teaspoon ground black pepper
- 1/2 tsp. curry powder
- 3/4 cup light mayonnaise
- dolor secatibero

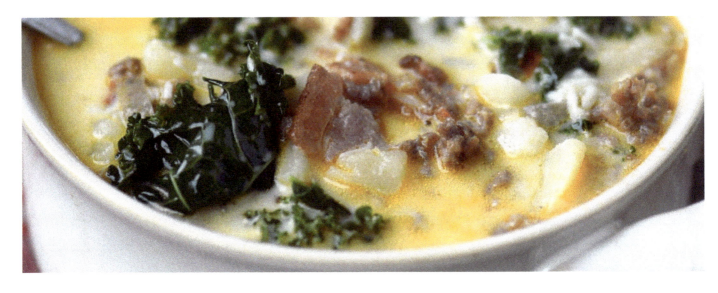

ZUPPA TOSCANA

TIME	COOKING	SERVE
25 MINS	60 MINS	3

Method

1. Cook that the Italian sausage and red pepper flakes in a pot on medium-high heat until crumbly, browned, with no longer pink, 10 to 15minutes. Drain and put aside.

2. Cook the bacon at the exact Dutch oven over moderate heat until crispy, about 10 minutes, drain, leaving a couple of tablespoons of drippings together with all the bacon at the bottom of the toaster. Stir in the garlic and onions cook until onions are tender and translucent, about five minutes.

3. Pour the chicken broth to the pot with the onion and bacon mix; contribute to a boil on high temperature. Add the berries, and boil until fork-tender, about 20 minutes. Reduce heat to moderate and stir in the cream and also the cooked sausage – heat throughout. Mix the lettuce to the soup before serving.

Nutrition

Per month: 554 carbs 32.6 grams fat 45.8 grams carbs 19.8 grams protein

Ingredients

- 1 lb. ground Italian sausage
- 1 1/4 tsp. crushed red pepper flakes
- 4 pieces bacon, cut into ½ inch bits
- 1 big onion, diced
- 1 tbsp. minced garlic
- 5 (13.75 oz.) can chicken broth
- 6 celery, thinly chopped
- 1 cup thick cream
- 1/4 bunch fresh spinach, tough stems removed

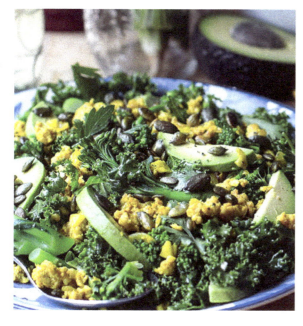

Turmeric Chicken & Kale Salad with
HONEY-LIME DRESSING

TIME **COOKING** **SERVE**

20 MINS 10 MINS 2

Method

1. Notes: when planning beforehand, dress the salad 10 minutes before serving. The chicken might be substituted with beef chopped, sliced prawns or fish. Vegetarians may use chopped mushrooms or cooked quinoa.

2. Heat the ghee or coconut oil at a tiny skillet pan above medium-high heat. Bring the onion and then sauté on moderate heat for 45 minutes, until golden. Insert the chicken blossom and garlic and simmer for 2-3 minutes on medium-high heat, breaking it all out.

3. Add the garlic, lime zest, lime juice, and salt and soda and cook stirring often, to get a further 3-4 minutes. Place the cooked mince aside.

4. As the chicken is cooking, add a little spoonful of water. Insert the broccoli and cook 2 minutes. Rinse under warm water and then cut into 3-4 pieces each.

5. Insert the pumpkin seeds into the skillet out of the toast and chicken over moderate heat for two minutes, stirring often to avoid burning. Season with a little salt. Set-aside. Raw pumpkin seeds will also be nice to utilize.

6. Put chopped spinach at a salad bowl and then pour over the dressing table. With the hands, massage and toss the carrot with the dressing table. This will dampen the lettuce, a lot similar to what citrus juice will not steak or fish Carpaccio— its "hamburgers" it marginally.

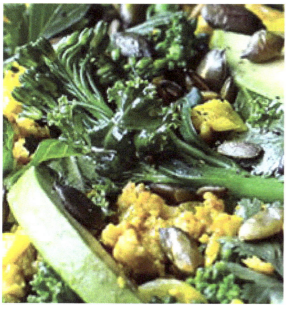

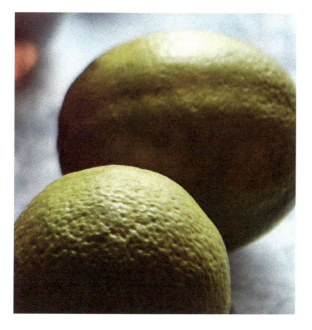

7. Finally, toss throughout the cooked chicken, broccoli, fresh herbs, pumpkin seeds, and avocado pieces.

Ingredients

- For your poultry
- 1 tsp. ghee or 1 tablespoon coconut oil
- 1/2 moderate brown onion, diced
- 250 300 grams / 9 oz. Chicken mince or pops upward chicken thighs
- 1 large garlic clove, finely-chopped
- 1 tsp. turmeric powder
- Optional 1teaspoon lime zest
- Juice of 1/2 lime
- 1/2 tsp. salt
- For your salad
- 6 broccoli 2 or two cups of broccoli florets
- 2 tbsp. pumpkin seeds (pepitas)
- 3 big kale leaves, stalks removed and sliced
- Optional 1/2 avocado, chopped
- Bunch of coriander leaves, chopped
- Couple of fresh parsley leaves, chopped
- For your dressing
- 3 tbsp. lime juice
- 1 small garlic clove, finely diced or grated
- 3 tbsp. extra virgin coconut oil (I used 1. tsp. avocado oil and 2 tbsp. Evo)
- 1 tsp. raw honey
- 1/2 tsp. whole grain or Dijon mustard
- 1/2 tsp. sea salt

Nutrition

Calories 166 Fats 13 g Carbohydrates 18 g Proteins 7 g

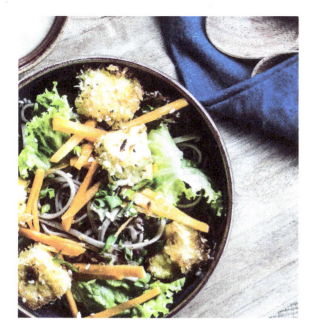

Buckwheat Noodles with Chicken Kale &

MISO DRESSING

TIME   **COOKING**   **SERVE**

15 MINS   15 MINS   2

Method

1. Bring a medium saucepan of water. Insert the kale and cook 1 minute, until slightly wilted. Remove and put aside but keep the water and put it back to boil. Insert the soba noodles and cook according to the package directions (usually about five minutes). Rinse under warm water and place aside.

2. Meanwhile, pan press the shiitake mushrooms at just a very little ghee or coconut oil (about a tsp.) for 23 minutes, until lightly browned on each side. Sprinkle with sea salt and then place aside.

3. In the exact skillet, warm olive oil ghee over medium-high heating system. Sauté onion and simmer for 2 3 minutes and add the chicken bits. Cook five minutes over medium heat, stirring a few days, you can put in the garlic, tamari sauce and just a tiny dab of water. Cook for a further 2-3 minutes, stirring often until chicken is cooked through.

4. Last, add the carrot and soba noodles and chuck throughout the chicken to heat up.

5. Mix the miso dressing and scatter on the noodles before eating; in this manner, you can retain dozens of enzymes that are beneficial at the miso.

7. Finally, toss throughout the cooked chicken, broccoli, fresh herbs, pumpkin seeds, and avocado pieces.

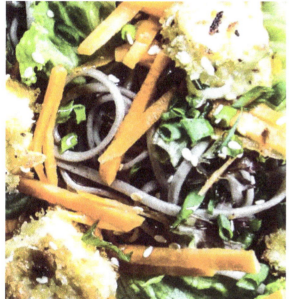

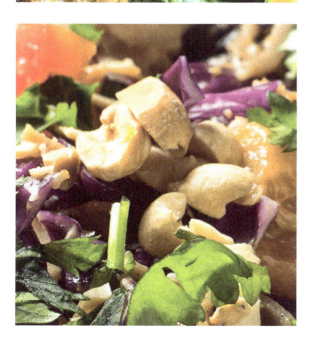

Ingredients

- For the noodles
- 2 3 handfuls of kale leaves (removed from the stem and fully trimmed)
- 150 g / 5 oz. buckwheat noodles (100 percent buckwheat, no wheat)
- 34 shiitake mushrooms, chopped
- 1 tsp. coconut oil or ghee
- 1 brown onion, finely diced
- 1 moderate free-range chicken, chopped or diced
- 1 red chili, thinly chopped (seeds out based on how hot you want it)
- 2 large garlic cloves, finely-chopped
- 23 tbsp. tamari sauce (fermented soy sauce)
- For your miso dressing
- 1 ½ tbsp. fresh organic miso
- 1 tbsp. tamari sauce
- 1 tbsp. peppermint oil
- 1 tbsp. lime or lemon juice
- 1 tsp. sesame oil (optional)

Nutrition

342 Calories

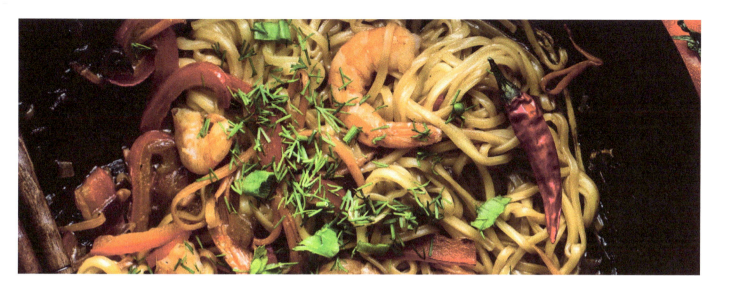

Asian King Prawn Stir Fry Together with

BUCKWHEAT NOODLES

TIME — 10 MINS

COOKING — 8 MINS

SERVE — 1

Ingredients

- 150g shelled raw king prawns, deveined
- Two tsp. tamari (it is possible to utilize soy sauce in the event that you aren't quitting gluten)
- Two tsp. extra virgin coconut oil, 75g soba (buckwheat noodles)
- 1 garlic clove, finely chopped
- 1 bird's-eye chili, finely chopped, 1 tsp. finely chopped ginger
- 20g red onions, chopped
- 40g celery, trimmed and chopped, 75g green beans, sliced
- 50g kale, approximately sliced, 100ml poultry inventory
- 5g lovage or celery leaves

Method

1. Heating a skillet on high heat, cook the prawns into 1 tsp. of this tamari and one tsp. of the oil 2--three minutes. Transfer the prawns into your plate. Wipe out the pan with kitchen paper, even because you are going to make use of it.

2. Cook the noodles in boiling water 8 minutes as directed on the package. Drain and put aside.

3. Meanwhile, squeeze the garlic, chili and ginger, red onion, celery, lettuce and beans at the rest of the oil over medium- high temperature for two-three minutes. Bring the stock and bring to the boil, then simmer for a moment or two, before the veggies have been cooked but still crunchy.

4. Insert both the prawns, noodles and lovage/celery leaves into the pan, then return to the boil and then remove from heat and serve.

Nutrition

340 Calories

DESSERT RECIPES

PHASE 1

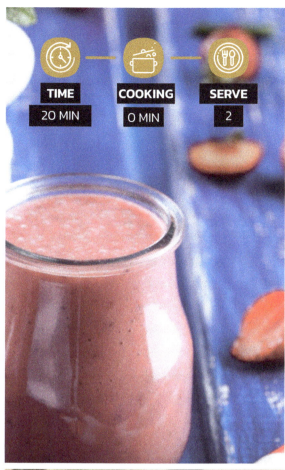

Creamy Strawberry & Cherry
SMOOTHY

TIME 20 MIN | **COOKING** 0 MIN | **SERVE** 2

Ingredients

- 100g 3½ oz. strawberries
- 75g 3oz. frozen pitted cherries
- 1 tablespoon plain full-fat yogurt
- 175mls 6fl oz. unsweetened soya milk
- 132 calories per serving

Method

1. Place all of the ingredients into a blender and process until smooth. Serve and enjoy.

Nutrition

Calories: 254.

Grape, Celery & Parsley
REVIVER

TIME 10 MINS | **COOKING** 0 MIN | **SERVE** 2

Ingredients

- 75g 3 oz. red grapes
- 3 sticks of celery
- 1 avocado, de-stoned and peeled
- 1 tablespoon fresh parsley
- ½ teaspoon Matcha powder
- 334 calories per serving

Method

1. Place all of the ingredients into a blender with enough water to cover them and blitz until smooth and creamy. Add crushed ice to make it even more refreshing.

Nutrition

Calories: 275

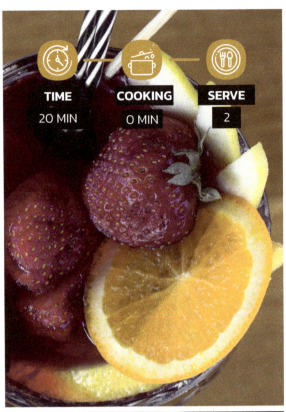

Strawberry & Citrus
BLEND

Ingredients

- 75g 3oz strawberries
- 1 apple, cored
- 1 orange, peeled
- ½ avocado, peeled and de-stoned
- ½ teaspoon Matcha powder
- Juice of 1 lime

Method

1. Place all of the ingredients into a blender with enough water to cover them and process until smooth.

Nutrition

272 calories per serving.

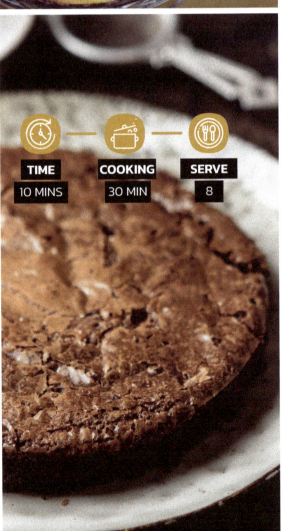

Chocolate Hazelnut
BROWNIE PIE

Ingredients

- ¾ cup of granulated Erythritol-based Sweetener
- 4 oz. of coarsely chopped unsweetened Chocolate
- 4 large eggs
- ½ cup of boiling Water
- 1 tsp. Vanilla extract
- 100g (1 cup) Hazelnut meal
- 1 stick (½ cups) unsalted Butter

Method

Heat the oven to 350° F. Grease a 9-inch ceramic pie pan or glass. Pulse the sweetener and the chopped chocolate in a food processor. Carefully pour in boiling water while the food processor is running on high until the chocolate becomes smooth and melted. Add the vanilla extract, butter, and eggs and process until it is well mixed. Fold in the hazelnut and process to make sure it well combined. Pour batter into greased pan and bake for 25-30 minutes so that the middle becomes somewhat wet but the sides becomes finely set. Take it out of the oven and cool. Refrigerate for 2 hours. Garnish with toasted hazelnuts and whipped cream.

Nutrition

Fat: 28.4g Carbs: 6.8g Protein: 7.3g Calories: 324

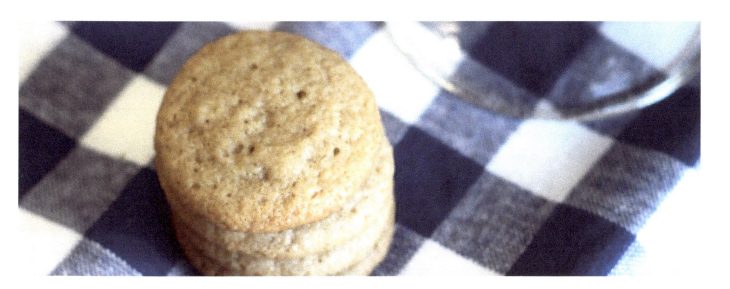

Slice-and-Bake

VANILLA WAFER

TIME — 10 MINS   **COOKING** — 15 MINS   **SERVE** — 2

Method

1. Beat the sweetener and butter using an electric mixer in a large bowl for 2 minutes until it becomes fluffy and light. Then beat in the salt, vanilla extract, coconut flour, and almond until thoroughly mixed.

2. Evenly spread the dough between two sheets of parchment or wax paper and wrap each portion into a size with a diameter of about 1½ inches. Then wrap in paper and refrigerate for 1-2 hours.

3. Heat the oven to 325° F and line a baking sheet using silicone baking mats or parchment paper. Slice the dough into ¼- inch slices using a sharp knife. Put the sliced dough on the baking sheets and make sure to leave a 1-inch space between wafers.

4. Place in the oven for about 5 minutes. Slightly flatten the cookies using a flat-bottomed glass. Bake for another 8-10 minutes.

Nutrition

Protein: 2.2g Fat: 9.3g Carbs: 2.5g Calories: 101

Ingredients

- 175g (1¾ cups) blanched Almond flour
- ½ cup granulated Erythritol-based Sweetener
- 1 stick (½ cup) unsalted softened Butter
- 2 tbsp. of Coconut flour
- ¼ tsp. of salt
- ½ tsp. of Vanilla extract

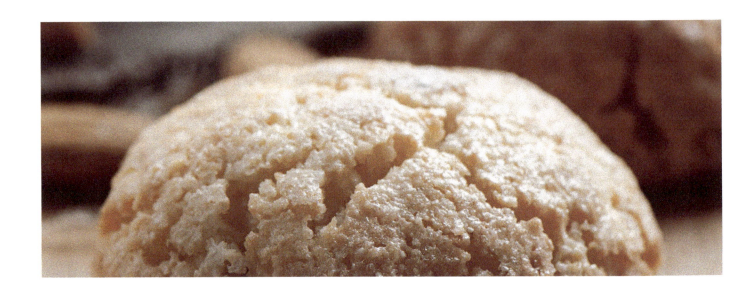

AMARETTI

TIME 15 MINS   **COOKING** 22 MINS   **SERVE** 2

Method

1. Heat the oven to 300° F and use parchment paper to line 2 baking sheets. Grease the parchment slightly.

2. Process the powdered sweetener, granulated sweetener, and sliced almonds in a food processor until it appears like coarse crumbs.

3. Beat the egg whites plus the salt and almond extracts using an electric mixer in a large bowl until they hold soft peaks. Fold in the almond mixture so that it becomes well combined.

4. Drop spoonful of the dough onto the prepared baking sheet and allow for a space of 1 inch between them. Press a sliced almond into the top of each cookie.

5. Bake in the oven for 22 minutes until the sides becomes brown. They will appear jellylike when they are taken out from the oven but will begin to be firms as it cools down.

Nutrition

Fat: 8.8g Carbs: 4.1g Protein: 5.3g Calories: 117

Ingredients

- ½ cup of granulated Erythritol-based Sweetener
- 165g (2 cups) sliced Almonds
- ¼ cup of powdered of Erythritol-based sweetener
- 4 large egg whites
- Pinch of salt
- ½ tsp. almond extract

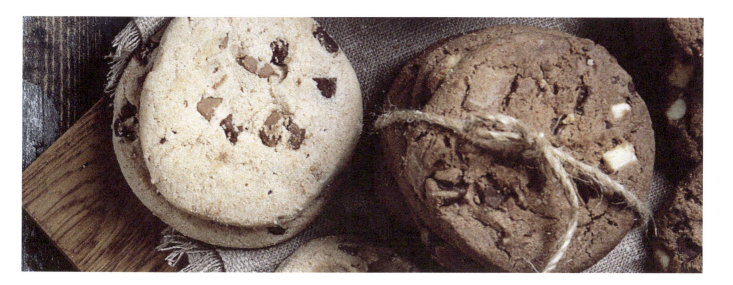

Peanut Butter

COOKIES FOR TWO

TIME 5 MINS   **COOKING** 12 MINS   **SERVE** 1

Method

1. Heat the oven to 325° F and line a baking sheet with a silicone baking mat or parchment paper.

2. Beat in the sweetener, butter, and peanut butter using an electric mixer in a small bowl until it is thoroughly mixed. Then beat in the vanilla extract and the egg.

3. Add the salt, baking powder, and peanut flour and mix until the dough clumps together. Cut the dough into two and shape each of them into a ball.

4. Position the dough ball into the coated baking sheets and flatten into a circular shape about ½ inches thick. Garnish the dough tops with a tsp. of chocolate chips. Gently press them into the dough to stick.

5. Bake for 10-12 minutes until golden brown.

Nutrition

: Fat: 13.2g Carbs: 5.7g

Protein: 4.9g Calories: 163

Ingredients

- 1½ tbsp. of creamy salted Peanut Butter
- 1 tbsp. of unsalted softened Butter
- 2 tsp. of lightly beaten egg
- 2 tbsp. of granulated Erythritol-based Sweetener
- ¼ tsp. of Vanilla extract
- 2 tbsp. of defatted Peanut flour
- Pinch of salt
- 2 tsp. of sugarless Chocolate Chips
- ⅛ Tsp. of baking powder

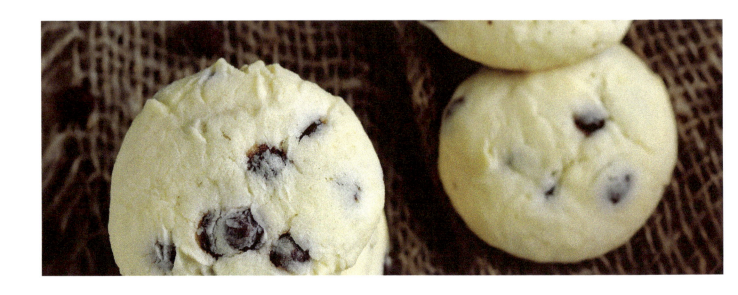

CREAM CHEESE COOKIES

TIME 15 MINS   **COOKING** 12 MINS   **SERVE** 6

Method

1. Heat the oven to 350°F and line with a silicone baking mat or parchment paper.

2. Beat the butter and cream cheese using an electric mixer in a large bowl until it appears smooth. Add the sweetener and keep beating. Beat in the vanilla extract and the egg.

3. Whisk in the salt, baking powder, and almond flour in a medium bowl. Add the flour mixture into the cream cheese and until well incorporated.

4. Drop the dough in spoonful onto the coated baking sheet. Flatten the cookies.

5. Bake for 10-12 minutes. Dust with powdered sweetener when cool.

Nutrition

Fat: 13.7g Carbs: 3.4g

Protein: 4.1g Calories: 154

Ingredients

- ¼ cup (½ stick) unsalted softened Butter
- ½ cup (4 oz.) of softened Cream Cheese
- 1 large egg at room temp
- ½ of cup granulated Erythritol-based Sweetener
- 150g (1½ cups) of blanched Almond flour
- 1 tsp. of baking Powder
- ½ tsp. of Vanilla extract
- Powdered Erythritol-based sweetener (for dusting)
- ¼ tsp. of salt

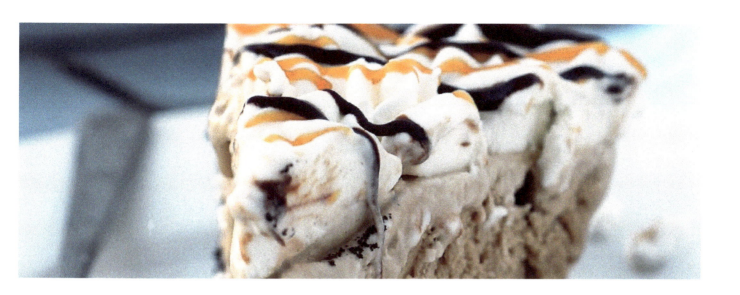

MOCHA CREAM PIE

TIME 15 MINS   **COOKING** 5 MINS   **SERVE** 10

Method

1. Grease a 9-inch glass pie pan or ceramic. Press the crust mixture evenly and firmly to the sides of the greased pan or its bottom. Refrigerate until the filling is prepared.

2. Pour the coffee in a small saucepan and add gelatin. Whisk thoroughly and then place over medium heat. Allow simmering, whisking from time to time to make sure the gelatin dissolves. Allow to cool for 20 minutes.

3. Add the vanilla extract, cocoa powder, sweetener, and the cream into a large bowl. Use an electric mixer to beat to that it holds stiff peaks.

4. Add gelatin mixture that has been cooled and then beat until it is well incorporated. Pour over the cooled crust and place in the refrigerator for 3 hours until it becomes firm.

Nutrition

Fat: 20.2g Carbs: 6.2g

Protein: 4.7g Calories: 218

Ingredients

- 1 cup strongly brewed Coffee at room temp
- 1 Easy Chocolate Pie Crust
- 1 cup heavy Whipping Cream
- 1½ tsp. of grass-fed Gelatin
- 1 tsp. of Vanilla extract
- ¼ cup Cocoa powder
- ½ cup powdered Erythritol-based Sweetener

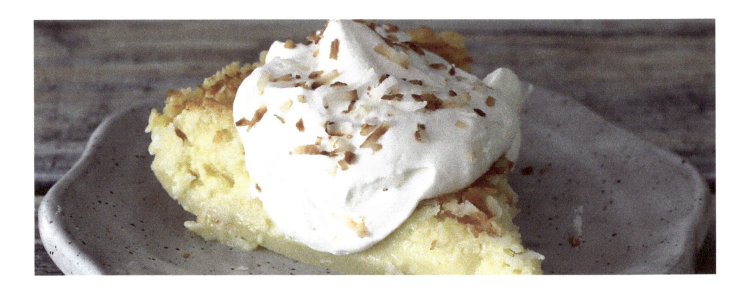

COCONUT CUSTARD PIE

TIME **COOKING** **SERVE**

10 MINS 50 MINS 8

Method

1. Heat the oven to 350° F and grease a 9-inch ceramic pie pan or glass.

2. Place the melted butter, eggs, coconut milk, sweetener, and cream in a blender. Blend well.

3. Add the vanilla extract, baking powder, salt, coconut flour, and a cup of shredded coconut. Continue blending.

4. Empty the mixture into the pie pan and sprinkle with the rest of the shredded coconut. Bake for 40-50 minutes and stop when the center is until jiggly but the sides are set.

5. Take out of the oven and allow it to cool for 30 minutes. Place in the refrigerator and allow staying for 2 hours before cutting it.

Nutrition

Fat: 29.5g Carbs: 6.7g

Protein: 5.3g Calories: 317

Ingredients

- 1 cup of heavy Whipping Cream
- ¾ cup of powdered Erythritol-based Sweetener
- ½ cup of full-fat Coconut Milk
- 4 large eggs
- ½ stick (¼ cup) of cooled, unsalted, melted butter
- 1¼ cups of unsweetened shredded coconut
- 3 tbsp. of Coconut flour
- ½ tsp. of baking powder
- ½ tsp. of Vanilla extract
- ¼ tsp. of salt

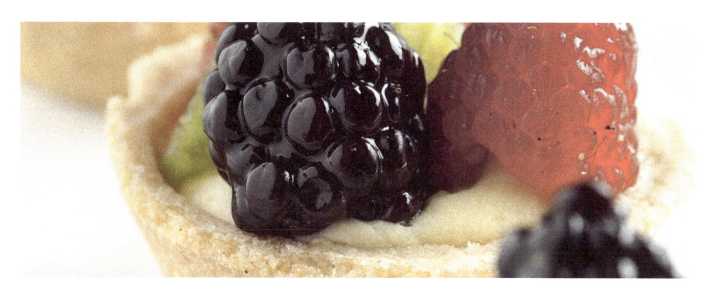

Dairy-Free

FRUIT TARTS

TIME — 15 MINS   **COOKING** — 15 MINS   **SERVE** — 2

Method

1. Grease two 4″ pans with detachable bottoms. Pour the shortbread mixture into pans and firmly press into the edges and bottom of each pan. Refrigerate for 15 minutes.

2. Loosen the crust carefully to remove from the pan.

3. Distribute the whipped cream between the tarts and evenly spread to the sides. Refrigerate for 1–2 hours to make it firm.

4. Use the berries and sprig of mint to garnish each of the tarts

Nutrition

Fat: 28.9g Carbs: 8.3g

Protein: 5.8g Calories: 306

Ingredients

- 1 cup Coconut Whipped Cream
- ½ Easy Shortbread Crust (dairy-free option)
- Fresh mint Sprigs
- ½ cup mixed fresh Berries

OTHER RECIPES

PHASE 1

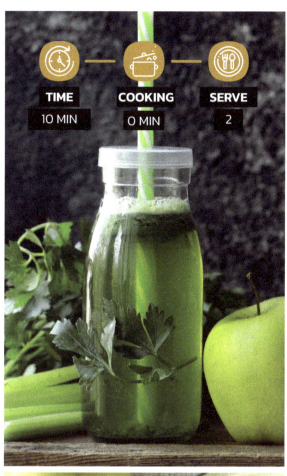

Apple & Celery JUICE

Ingredients
- 4 large green apples, cored and sliced
- 4 celery stalks
- 1 lemon, peeled

Method
1. Add all ingredients into a juicer and extract the juice according to the manufacturer's method.
2. Pour into 2 glasses and serve immediately.

Nutrition
Calories 240, Total Fat 0.9 g, Saturated Fat 0 g, Cholesterol 0 mg, Protein 1.5 g

TIME 10 MIN | **COOKING** 0 MIN | **SERVE** 2

Broccoli, Apple, & ORANGE JUICE

Ingredients
- 2 broccoli stalks, chopped
- 2 large green apples, cored and sliced
- 3 large oranges, peeled and sectioned
- 4 tablespoons fresh parsley

Method
1. Add all ingredients into a juicer and extract the juice according to the manufacturer's method.
2. Pour into 2 glasses and serve immediately.

Nutrition
Calories 254, Total Fat 0.8 g, Saturated Fat 0.1 g, Protein 3.8 g

TIME 10 MINS | **COOKING** 0 MIN | **SERVE** 2

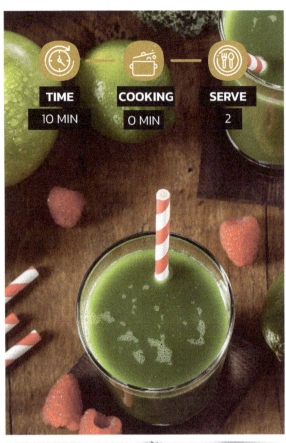

Green Fruit JUICE

Ingredients

- 3 large kiwis, peeled and chopped
- 3 large green apples, cored and sliced
- 2 cups seedless green grapes
- 2 teaspoons fresh lime juice

Method

1. Add all ingredients into a juicer and extract the juice according to the manufacturer's method.

2. Pour into 2 glasses and serve immediately.

Nutrition

Calories 304, Total Fat 2.2 g, Saturated Fat 0 g, Protein 6.2 g

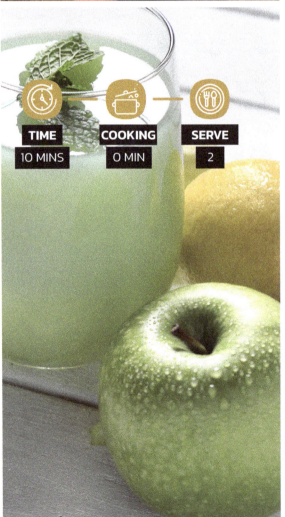

Kale & Fruit JUICE

Ingredients

- 2 large green apples, cored and sliced
- 2 large pears, cored and sliced
- 3 cups fresh kale leaves
- 3 celery stalks
- 1 lemon, peeled

Method

1. Add all ingredients into a juicer and extract the juice according to the manufacturer's method.

2. Pour into 2 glasses and serve immediately.

Nutrition

Calories 293 Total Fat 0.8 g Saturated Fat 0 g Cholesterol 0 mg Protein 4.6 g

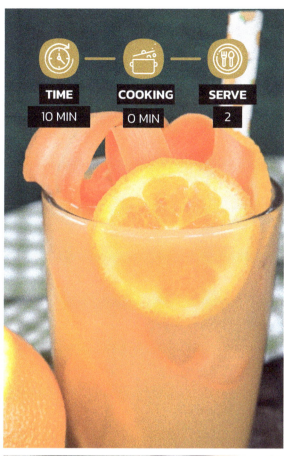

Kale, Carrot, & Grapefruit
JUICE

TIME 10 MIN | **COOKING** 0 MIN | **SERVE** 2

Ingredients

- 3 cups fresh kale
- 2 large Granny Smith apples, cored and sliced
- 2 medium carrots, peeled and chopped
- 2 medium grapefruit, peeled and sectioned
- 1 teaspoon fresh lemon juice

Method

1. Add all ingredients into a juicer and extract the juice according to the manufacturer's method.

2. Pour into 2 glasses and serve immediately.

Nutrition

Calories 232, Total Fat 0.6 g, Saturated Fat 0 ,g Cholesterol 0 mg, Protein 4.9 g

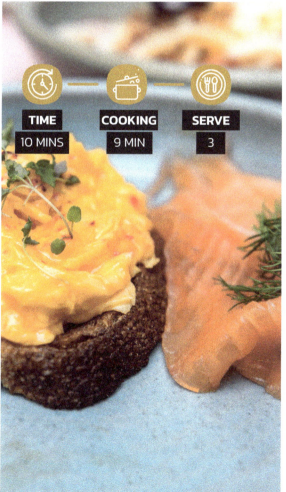

Smoked Salmon &
KALE SCRAMBLE

TIME 10 MINS | **COOKING** 9 MIN | **SERVE** 3

Ingredients

- 2 cups fresh kale, tough ribs removed and chopped finely
- 1 tablespoon coconut oil
- Ground black pepper, to taste
- ½ cup smoked salmon, crumbled
- 4 eggs, beaten

Method

1. In a wok, melt the coconut oil over high heat and cook the kale with black pepper for about 3–4 minutes.

2. Stir in the smoked salmon and reduce the heat to medium.

3. Add the eggs and cook for about 3–4 minutes, stirring frequently.

4. Serve immediately.

Nutrition

Calories 257, Total Fat 17 g, Saturated Fat 8.9 g ,Cholesterol 335 mg, Protein 19.3 g

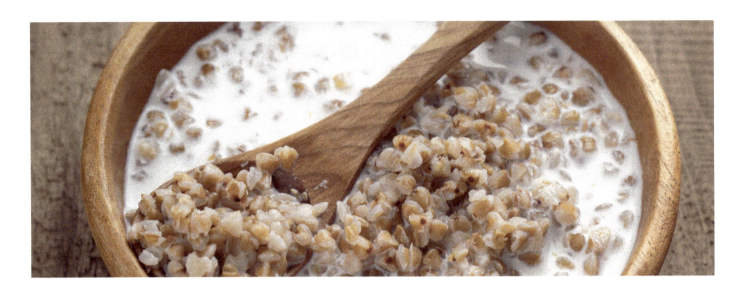

BUCKWHEAT GRANOLA

TIME **COOKING** **SERVE**
15 MINS 30 MINS 10

Method

1. Preheat your oven to 350°F.

2. In a bowl, place the buckwheat groats, coconut flakes, pumpkin seeds, almonds, and spices, and mix well.

3. In another bowl, add the banana and with a fork, mash well.

4. Add to the buckwheat mixture maple syrup and oil, and mix until well combined.

5. Transfer the mixture onto the prepared baking sheet and spread in an even layer.

6. Bake for about 25–30 minutes, stirring once halfway through.

7. Remove the baking sheet from oven and set aside to cool.

Nutrition

Calories 252, Total Fat 14.3 g, Saturated Fat 3.7 g,

Cholesterol 0 mg, Protein 7.6 g

Ingredients

- 2 cups raw buckwheat groats
- ¾ cup pumpkin seeds
- ¾ cup almonds, chopped
- 1 cup unsweetened coconut flakes
- 1 teaspoon ground cinnamon
- 1 teaspoon ground ginger
- 1 ripe banana, peeled
- 2 tablespoons maple syrup
- 2 tablespoons olive oil

APPLE PANCAKES

TIME
15 MINS

COOKING
24 MINS

SERVE
6

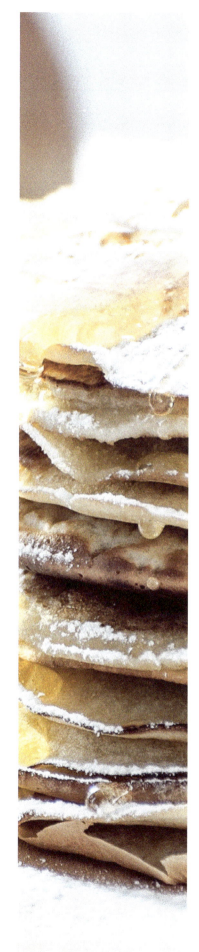

Method

1. In a bowl, place the flour, coconut sugar, and cinnamon, and mix well.

2. In another bowl, place the almond milk and egg and beat until well combined.

3. Now, place the flour mixture and mix until well combined.

4. Fold in the grated apples.

5. Heat a lightly greased non-stick wok over medium-high heat.

6. Add desired amount of mixture and with a spoon, spread into an even layer.

7. Cook for 1–2 minutes on each side.

8. Repeat with the remaining mixture.

9. Serve warm with the drizzling of honey.

Nutrition

Calories 93, Total Fat 2.1 g, Saturated Fat 1 g, Cholesterol 27 mg, Sugar 12.1 g, Protein 2.5 g

Ingredients

- ½ cup buckwheat flour
- 2 tablespoons coconut sugar
- 1 teaspoon baking powder
- ½ teaspoon ground cinnamon
- 1/3 cup unsweetened almond milk
- 1 egg, beaten lightly
- 2 granny smith apples, peeled, cored, and grated

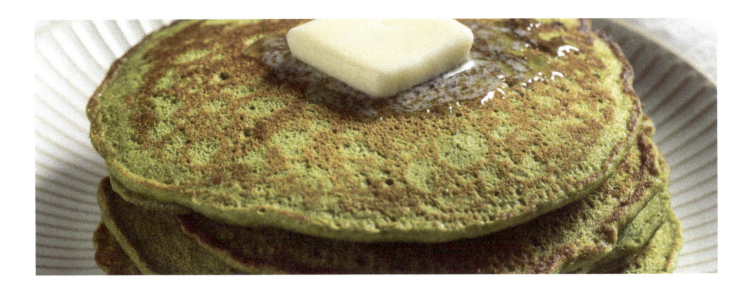

MATCHA PANCAKES

TIME 15 MINS   **COOKING** 24 MINS   **SERVE** 6

Method

1. In a bowl, add the flax meal and warm water and mix well. Set aside for about 5 minutes.

2. In another bowl, place the flours, Matcha powder, baking powder, and salt, and mix well.

3. In the bowl of flax meal mixture, place the almond milk, oil, and vanilla extract, and beat until well combined.

4. Now, place the flour mixture and mix until a smooth textured mixture is formed.

5. Heat a lightly greased non-stick wok over medium-high heat.

6. Add desired amount of mixture and with a spoon, spread into an even layer.

7. Cook for about 2–3 minutes.

8. Carefully, flip the side and cook for about 1 minute.

9. Repeat with the remaining mixture. Serve warm with the drizzling of honey

Nutrition

Calories 232 Total Fat 4.6 g Saturated Fat 0.6 g

Cholesterol 0 mg Protein 6 g

Ingredients

- 2 tablespoons flax meal
- 5 tablespoons warm water
- 1 cup spelt flour
- 1 cup buckwheat flour
- 1 tablespoon Matcha powder
- 1 tablespoon baking powder
- Pinch of salt
- ¾ cup unsweetened almond milk
- 1 tablespoon olive oil
- 1 teaspoon vanilla extract
- 1/3 cup raw honey

KALE & MUSHROOM FRITTATA

TIME 15 MINS **COOKING** 30 MINS **SERVE** 5

Method

1. Preheat oven to 350°F.

2. In a large bowl, place the eggs, coconut milk, salt, and black pepper, and beat well. Set aside.

3. In a large ovenproof wok, heat the oil over medium heat and sauté the onion and garlic for about 3–4 minutes.

4. Add the squash, kale, bell pepper, salt, and black pepper, and cook for about 8–10 minutes.

5. Stir in the mushrooms and cook for about 3–4 minutes.

6. Add the kale and cook for about 5 minutes.

7. Place the egg mixture on top evenly and cook for about 4 minutes, without stirring.

8. Transfer the wok in the oven and bake for about 12–15 minutes or until desired doneness.

9. Remove from the oven and place the frittata side for about 3–5 minutes before serving.

10. Cut into desired sized wedges and serve.

Nutrition

Calories 151 Total Fat 10.2 g Saturated Fat 2.6 g Cholesterol 262 mg Protein 10.3 g

Ingredients

- 8 eggs
- ½ cup unsweetened almond milk
- Salt and ground black pepper, to taste
- 1 tablespoon olive oil
- 1 onion, chopped
- 1 garlic clove, minced
- 1 cup fresh mushrooms, chopped
- 1½ cups fresh kale, tough ribs removed and chopped

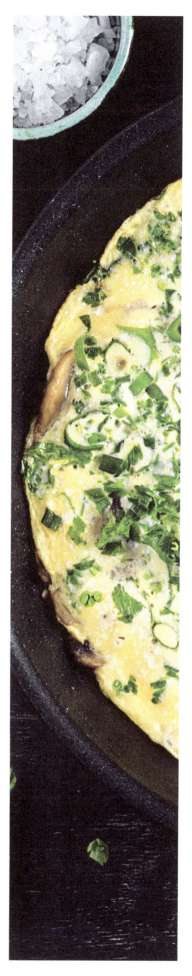

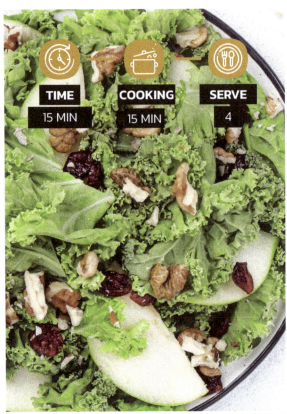

Kale, Apple, & Cranberry SALAD

TIME 15 MIN | **COOKING** 15 MIN | **SERVE** 4

Ingredients

- 6 cups fresh baby kale
- 3 large apples, cored and sliced
- ¼ cup unsweetened dried cranberries
- ¼ cup almonds, sliced
- 2 tablespoons extra-virgin olive oil, 1 tablespoon raw honey
- Salt and ground black pepper, to taste

Method

1. In a salad bowl, place all the ingredients and toss to coat well.
2. Serve immediately.

Nutrition

Calories 253, Total Fat 10.3 g, Saturated Fat 1.2 g, Cholesterol 0. mg Protein 4.7 g

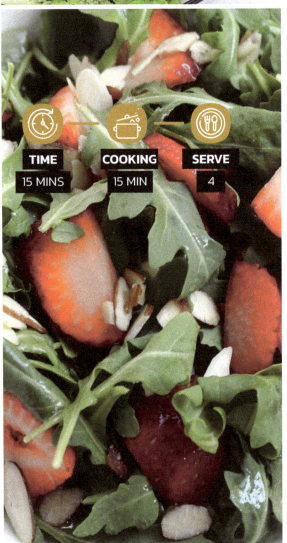

Arugula, Strawberry, & ORANGE SALAD

TIME 15 MINS | **COOKING** 15 MIN | **SERVE** 4

Ingredients

Salad

- 6 cups fresh baby arugula
- 1½ cups fresh strawberries, hulled and sliced
- 2 oranges, peeled and segmented

Dressing

- 2 tablespoons fresh lemon juice, 1 tablespoon raw honey
- 2 teaspoons extra-virgin olive oil, 1 teaspoon Dijon mustard
- Salt and ground black pepper, to taste

Method

1. For salad: in a salad bowl, place all ingredients and mix.
2. For dressing: place all ingredients in another bowl and beat until well combined.
3. Place dressing on top of salad and toss to coat well.
4. Serve immediately.

Nutrition

Calories 107 Total Fat 2.9 g Saturated Fat 0.4 g Cholesterol 0 mg Protein 2.1 g

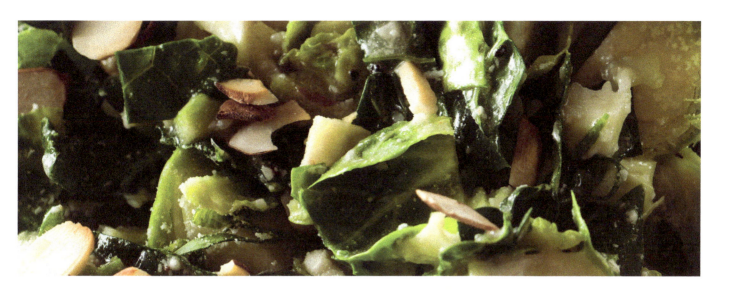

BEEF & KALE SALAD

TIME
15 MINS

COOKING
8 MINS

SERVE
2

Method

1. For steak: in a large heavy-bottomed wok, heat the oil over high heat and cook the steaks with salt and black pepper for about 3–4 minutes per side.

2. Transfer the steaks onto a cutting board for about 5 minutes before slicing.

3. For salad: place all ingredients in a salad bowl and mix.

4. For dressing: place all ingredients in another bowl and beat until well combined.

5. Cut the steaks into desired sized slices against the grain.

6. Place the salad onto each serving plate.

7. Top each plate with steak slices.

8. Drizzle with dressing and serve.

Nutrition

Calories 262 Total Fat 12 g Saturated Fat 1.6 g Protein 25.2 g

Ingredients

- Steak
- 2 teaspoons olive oil
- 2 (4-ounce) strip steaks
- Salt and ground black pepper, to tast
- Salad
- ¼ cup carrot, peeled and shredded
- ¼ cup cucumber, peeled, seeded, and sliced, ¼ cup radish, sliced
- ¼ cup cherry tomatoes, halved
- 3 cups fresh kale, tough ribs removed and chopped
- Dressing
- 1 tablespoon extra-virgin olive oil, Salt and ground black pepper, to taste
- 1 tablespoon fresh lemon juice

BREAKFAST RECIPES

PHASE 2

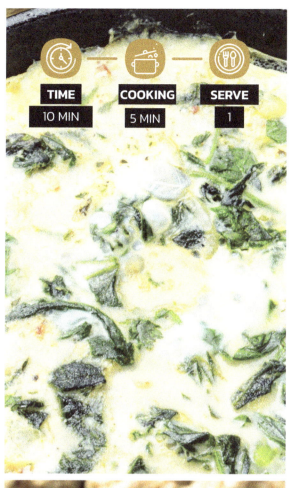

TIME 10 MIN | **COOKING** 5 MIN | **SERVE** 1

Green
OMELETTE

Ingredients

- 2 large eggs, at room temperature
- 1 shallot, peeled and chopped
- Handful arugula
- 3 sprigs of parsley, chopped
- 1 tsp. extra virgin olive oil
- Salt and black pepper

Method

Beat the eggs in a small bowl and set aside, sauté the shallot for 5 minutes with a bit of the oil, on low-medium heat. Pour the eggs in the pans, stirring the mixture for just a second. The eggs on a medium heat, and tip the pan just enough to let the loose egg run underneath after about one minute on the burner. Add the greens, herbs, and the seasonings to the top side as it is still soft. TIP: You do not even have to flip it, as you can just cook the egg slowly egg as is well (being careful as to not burn).

TIP: Another option is to put it into an oven to broil for 3-5 minutes (checking to make sure it is only until it is golden but burned).

Nutrition

Calories: 234.

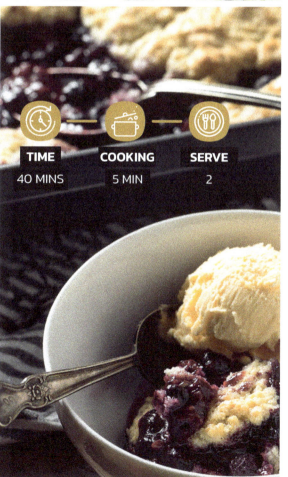

TIME 40 MINS | **COOKING** 5 MIN | **SERVE** 2

Berry Oat Breakfast
COBBLER

Ingredients

- 2 cups of oats/flakes that are ready without cooking
- 1 cup of blackcurrants without the stems
- 1 teaspoon of honey (or ¼ teaspoon of raw sugar)
- ½ cup of water (add more or less by testing the pan)
- 1 cup of plain yogurt (or soy or coconut)

Method

1. Boil the berries, honey and water and then turn it down on low. Put in a glass container in a refrigerator until it is cool and set (about 30 minutes or more)

2. When ready to eat, scoop the berries on top of the oats and yogurt. Serve immediately.

Nutrition

Calories: 241.

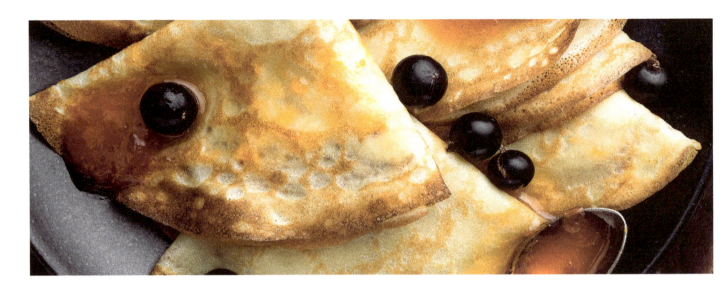

Pancakes with Apples and BLACKCURRANTS

TIME 30 MINS   **COOKING** 10 MINS   **SERVE** 4

Method

1. Place the ingredients for the topping in a small pot simmer, stirring frequently for about 10 minutes until it cooks down and the juices are released.

2. Take the dry ingredients and mix in a bowl. After, add the apples and the milk a bit at a time (you may not use it all), until it is a batter. Stiffly whisk the egg whites and then gently mix them into the pancake batter. Set aside in the refrigerator.

3. Pour a one quarter of the oil onto a flat pan or flat griddle, and when hot, pour some of the batter into it in a pancake shape. When the pancakes start to have golden brown edges and form air bubbles, they may be ready to be gently flipped.

4. Test to be sure the bottom can life away from the pan before actually flipping. Repeat for the next three pancakes. Top each pancake with the berries.

Nutrition

Calories: 337

Ingredients

- 2 apples, cut into small chunks
- 2 cups of quick cooking oats
- 1 cup flour of your choice
- 1 tsp. baking powder
- 2 tbsp. raw sugar, coconut sugar, or 2 tbsp. honey that is warm and easy to distribute
- 2 egg whites
- 1 ¼ cups of milk (or soy/rice/coconut)
- 2 tsp. extra virgin olive oil
- A dash of salt
- For the berry topping:
- 1 cup blackcurrants, washed and stalks removed
- 3 tbsp. water (may use less)
- 2 tbsp. sugar (see above for types)

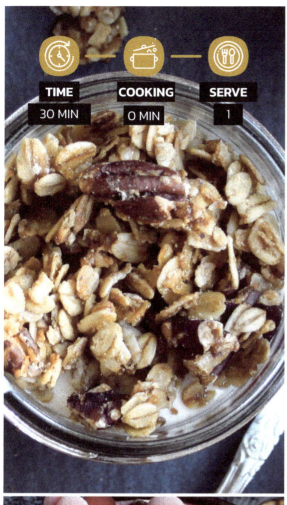

GRANOLA
The Sirt Way

TIME 30 MIN | **COOKING** 0 MIN | **SERVE** 1

Ingredients

- 1 cup buckwheat puffs
- 1 cup buckwheat flakes (ready to eat type, but not whole buckwheat that needs to be cooked) ½ cup coconut flakes
- ½ cup Medjool dates, without pits, chopped into smaller, bite-sized pieces
- 1 cup of cacao nibs or very dark chocolate chips
- 1/2 cup walnuts, chopped
- 1 cup strawberries chopped and without stem 1 cup plain Greek, or coconut or soy yogurt.

Method

1. Mix, without yogurt and strawberry toppings

2. You can store for up to a week, store in an airtight container. Add toppings (even different berries or different yogurt.

3. You can even use the berry toppings as you will learn how to make from other recipes.

Nutrition

Calories: 235.

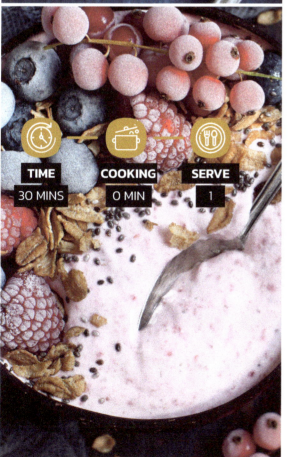

Summer Berry
SMOOTHIE

TIME 30 MINS | **COOKING** 0 MIN | **SERVE** 1

Ingredients

- 50g (2oz) blueberries
- 50g (2oz) strawberries
- 25g (1oz) blackcurrants
- 25g (1oz) red grapes
- 1 carrot, peeled
- 1 orange, peeled
- Juice of 1 lime

Method

1. Place all of the ingredients into a blender and cover them with water. Blitz until smooth. You can also add some crushed ice and a mint leaf to garnish.

Nutrition

Calories: 300.

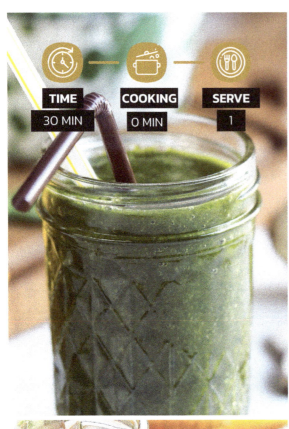

Mango, Celery & Ginger
SMOOTHIE

Ingredients

- 1 stalk of celery
- 50g (2oz) kale
- 1 apple, cored
- 50g (2oz) mango, peeled, de-stoned and chopped
- 2.5cm (1 inch) chunk of fresh ginger root, peeled and chopped

Method

1. Put all the ingredients into a blender with some water and blitz until smooth. Add ice to make your smoothie really refreshing.

Nutrition

Calories: 275.

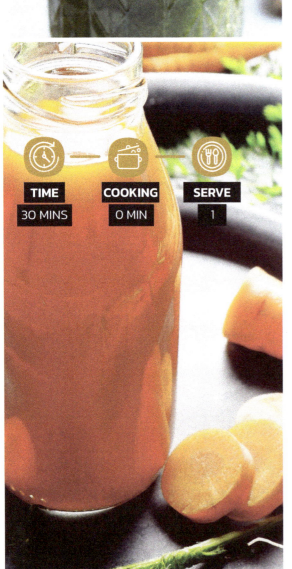

Orange, Carrot & Kale
SMOOTHIE

Ingredients

- 1 carrot, peeled
- 1 orange, peeled
- 1 stick of celery
- 1 apple, cored
- 50g (2oz) kale
- ½ teaspoon Matcha powder

Method

1. Place all of the ingredients into a blender and add in enough water to cover them. Process until smooth, serve and enjoy.

Nutrition

Calories: 279.

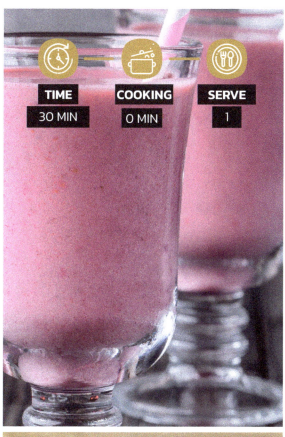

Creamy Strawberry & Cherry
SMOOTHIE

TIME 30 MIN | **COOKING** 0 MIN | **SERVE** 1

Ingredients
- 100g (3½ oz.) strawberries
- 75g (3oz) frozen pitted cherries
- 1 tablespoon plain full-fat yogurt
- 175mls (6fl oz.) unsweetened soya milk

Method
1. Place all of the ingredients into a blender and process until smooth. Serve and enjoy.

Nutrition
Calories: 280.

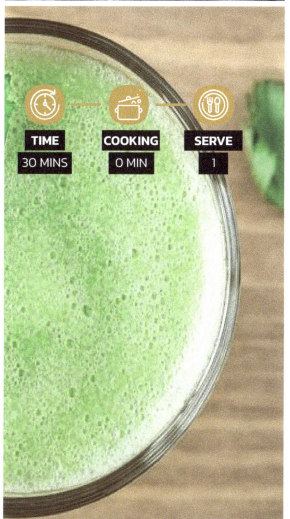

Grape, Celery & Parsley
REVIVER

TIME 30 MINS | **COOKING** 0 MIN | **SERVE** 1

Ingredients
- 75g (3oz) red grapes
- 3 sticks of celery
- 1 avocado, de-stoned and peeled
- 1 tablespoon fresh parsley
- ½ teaspoon Matcha powder

Method
1. Place all of the ingredients into a blender with enough water to cover them and blitz until smooth and creamy. Add crushed ice to make it even more refreshing.

Nutrition
Calories: 230.

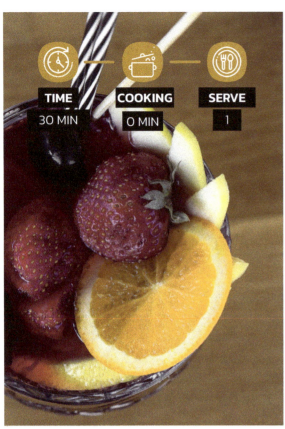

Strawberry & Citrus
BLEND

TIME 30 MIN | **COOKING** 0 MIN | **SERVE** 1

Ingredients

- 75g (3oz) strawberries
- 1 apple, cored
- 1 orange, peeled
- ½ avocado, peeled and de-stoned
- ½ teaspoon Matcha powder
- Juice of 1 lime

Method

1. Place all of the ingredients into a blender with enough water to cover them and process until smooth.

Nutrition

Calories: 250.

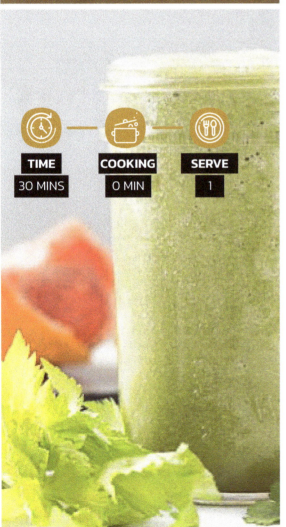

Grapefruit & Celery
BLAST

TIME 30 MINS | **COOKING** 0 MIN | **SERVE** 1

Ingredients

- 1 grapefruit, peeled
- 2 stalks of celery
- 50g (2oz) kale
- ½ teaspoon Matcha powder

Method

1. Place all the ingredients into a blender with enough water to cover them and blitz until smooth.

Nutrition

Calories: 286.

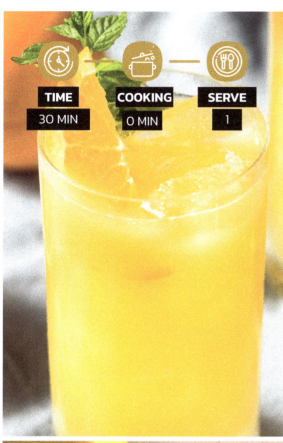

Orange & Celery
CRUSH

TIME 30 MIN | **COOKING** 0 MIN | **SERVE** 1

Ingredients

- 1 carrot, peeled
- 3 stalks of celery
- 1 orange, peeled
- ½ teaspoon Matcha powder
- Juice of 1 lime

Method

1. Place all of the ingredients into a blender with enough water to cover them and blitz until smooth.

Nutrition

Calories: 274.

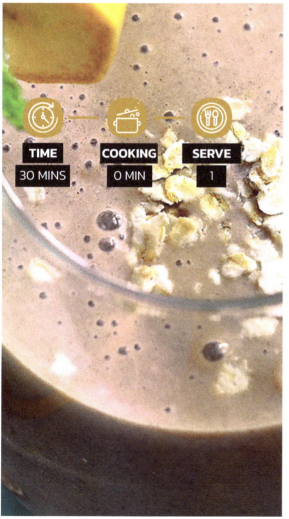

Tropical Chocolate
DELIGHT

TIME 30 MINS | **COOKING** 0 MIN | **SERVE** 1

Ingredients

- 1 mango, peeled & de-stoned
- 75g (3oz) fresh pineapple, chopped
- 50g (2oz) kale
- 25g (1oz) rocket
- 1 tablespoon 100% cocoa powder or cacao nibs
- 150mls (5fl oz.) coconut milk

Method

1. Place all of the ingredients into a blender and blitz until smooth. You can add a little water if it seems too thick.

Nutrition

Calories: 288.

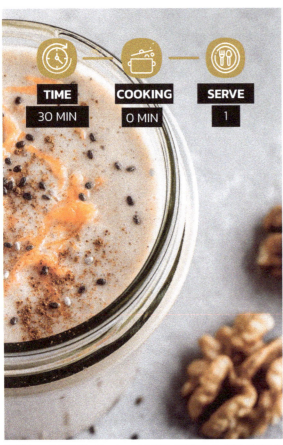

Walnut & Spiced Apple
TONIC

Ingredients

- 6 walnuts halves
- 1 apple, cored
- 1 banana
- ½ teaspoon Matcha powder
- ½ teaspoon cinnamon
- Pinch of ground nutmeg

Method

1. Place all of the ingredients into a blender and add sufficient water to cover them, blitz until smooth and creamy.

Nutrition

Calories: 258.

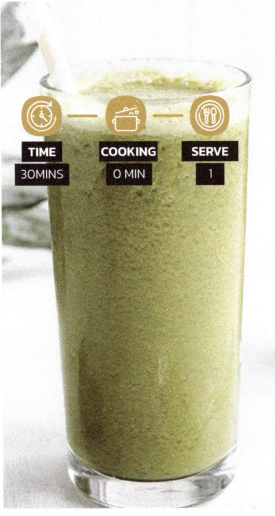

Pineapple & Cucumber
SMOOTHIE

Ingredients

- 50g (2oz) cucumber
- 1 stalk of celery
- 2 slices of fresh pineapple
- 2 sprigs of parsley
- ½ teaspoon Matcha powder
- Squeeze of lemon juice

Method

1. Place all of the ingredients into blender with enough water to cover them and blitz until smooth.

Nutrition

Calories: 260.

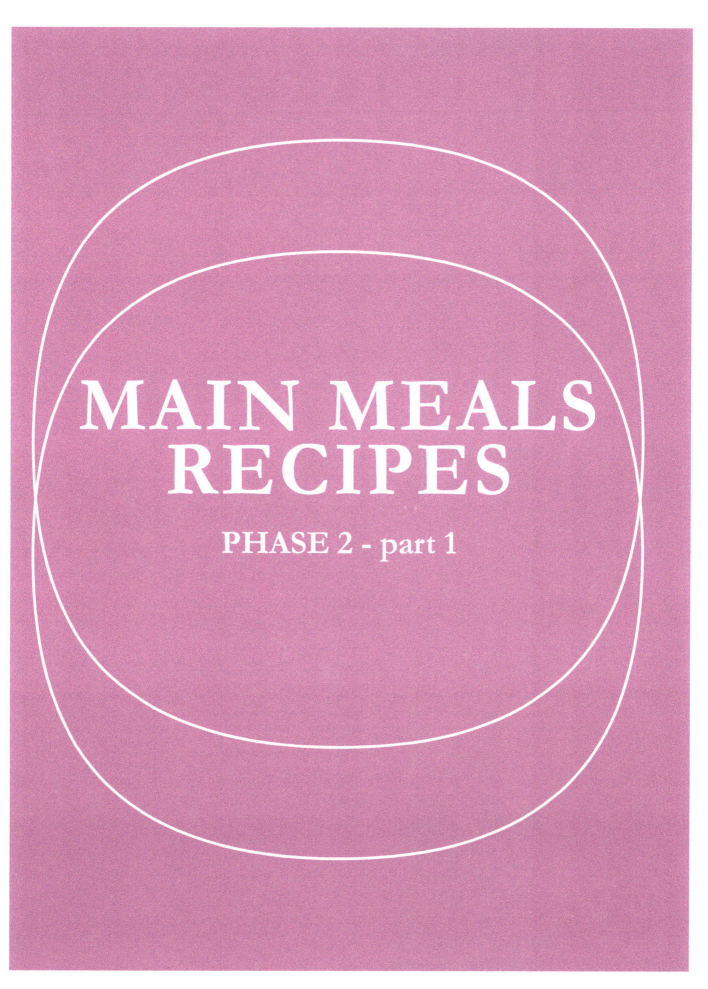

MAIN MEALS RECIPES

PHASE 2 - part 1

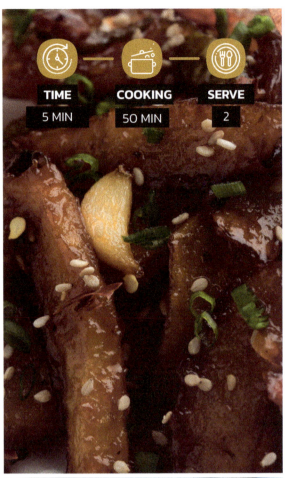

TIME 5 MIN — COOKING 50 MIN — SERVE 2

Honey Chili
SQUASH

Ingredients

- 2 red onions, roughly chopped 2.5cm
- 1-inch chunk of ginger root, finely chopped
- 2 cloves of garlic
- 2 bird's-eye chilies, finely chopped
- 1 butternut squash, peeled and chopped
- 100 ml 3½ fl. oz. vegetable stock broth
- 1 tablespoon olive oil
- Juice of 1 orange
- Juice of 1 lime
- 2 teaspoons honey

Method

1. Warm the oil into a pan and add in the red onions, squash chunks, chilies, garlic, ginger and honey. Cook for 3 minutes. Squeeze in the lime and orange juice. Pour in the stock broth), orange and lime juice and cook for 15 minutes until tender.

Nutrition

Calories: 118 Cal per serving.

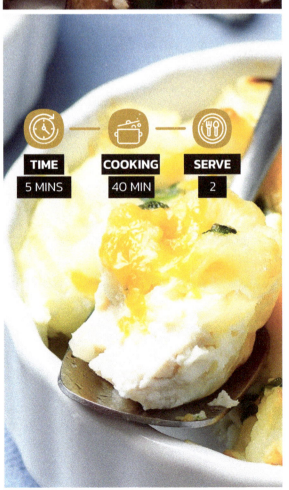

TIME 5 MINS — COOKING 40 MIN — SERVE 2

Chicken & Bean
CASSEROLE

Ingredients

- 400g 14oz chopped tomatoes
- 400g 14 oz. tinned cannellini beans or haricot beans
- 8 chicken thighs, skin removed
- 2 carrots, peeled and finely chopped
- 2 red onions, chopped
- 4 sticks of celery
- 4 large mushrooms
- 2 red peppers bell peppers, deseeded and chopped
- 1 clove of garlic
- 2 tablespoons soy sauce
- 1 tablespoon olive oil
- 1.75 liters 3 pints chicken stock broth

Method

1. Heat the olive oil in a saucepan, add the garlic and onions and cook for 5 minutes. Add in the chicken and cook for 5 minutes then add the carrots, cannellini beans, celery, red peppers bell peppers and mushrooms. Pour in the stock broth soy sauce and tomatoes. Bring it to the boil, reduce the heat and simmer for 45 minutes. Serve with rice or new potatoes.

Nutrition

509 calories per serving

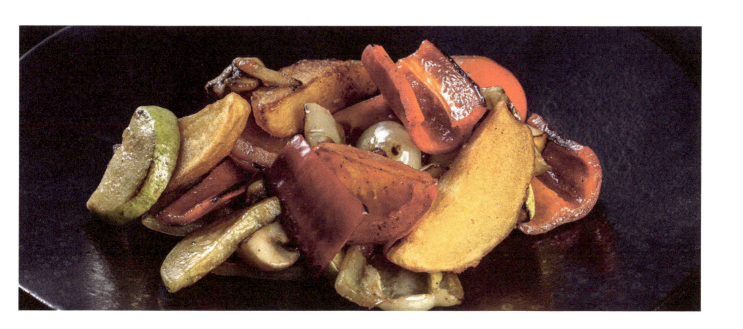

ROAST BALSAMIC VEGETABLES

TIME 5 MINS   **COOKING** 45 MINS   **SERVE** 2

Ingredients

- 4 tomatoes, chopped
- 2 red onions, chopped
- 3 sweet potatoes, peeled and chopped
- 100g 3½ oz. red chicory or if unavailable, use yellow
- 100g 3½ oz. kale, finely chopped
- 300g 11oz potatoes, peeled and chopped
- 5 stalks of celery, chopped
- 1 bird's-eye chili, de-seeded and finely chopped
- 2 tablespoons fresh parsley, chopped
- 2 tablespoons fresh coriander cilantro chopped
- 3 tablespoons olive oil
- 2 tablespoons balsamic vinegar 1 teaspoon mustard
- Sea salt
- Freshly ground black pepper

Method

1. Place the olive oil, balsamic, mustard, parsley and coriander cilantro into a bowl and mix well. Toss all the remaining ingredients into the dressing and season with salt and pepper. Transfer the vegetables to an ovenproof dish and cook in the oven at 200C/400F for 45 minutes.

Nutrition

310 calories per serving.

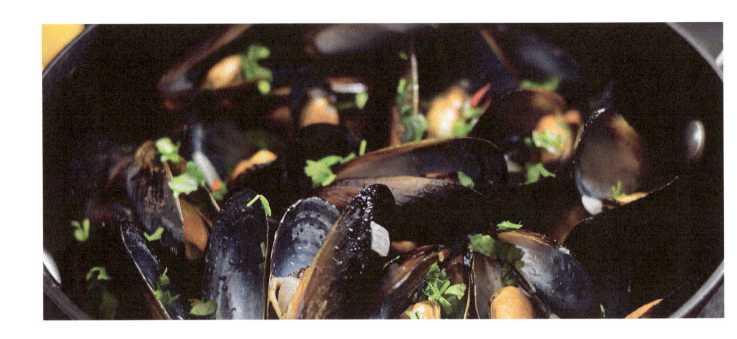

Mussels in Red

WINE SAUCE

TIME 5 MINS   **COOKING** 50 MINS   **SERVE** 2

Method

1. Wash the mussels, remove their beards and set them aside. Heat the butter in a large saucepan and add in the red wine. Reduce the heat and add the parsley, chives, chili and garlic whilst stirring. Add in the tomatoes, lemon juice and mussels. Cover the saucepan and cook for 2–3 minutes. Remove the saucepan from the heat and take out any mussels which haven't opened and discard them. Serve and eat immediately.

Nutrition

Calories: 364 per serving.

Ingredients

- 800g 2lb mussels
- 2 x 400g 14 oz. tins of chopped tomatoes
- 25g 1oz butter
- 1 tablespoon fresh chives, chopped
- 1 tablespoon fresh parsley, chopped
- 1 bird's-eye chili, finely chopped
- 4 cloves of garlic, crushed
- 400 ml 14fl. oz. red wine
- Juice of 1 lemon

MAIN MEALS RECIPES

PHASE 2 - part 2

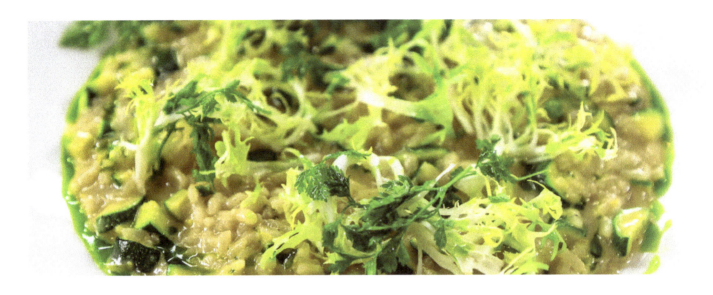

COURGETTE RISOTTO

TIME 10 MINS

COOKING 5 MINS

SERVE 8

Method

1. Place a large heavy bottomed pan over medium heat. Add oil. When the oil is heated, add onion and sauté until translucent.

2. Stir in the tomatoes and cook until soft.

3. Next stir in the rice and rosemary, mix well.

4. Add half the stock and cook until dry. Stir frequently.

5. Add remaining stock and cook for 3-4 minutes.

6. Add courgette and peas and cook until rice is tender. Add salt and pepper to taste.

7. Stir in the basil. Let it sit for 5 minutes.

Nutrition

Calories 406 Fats 5 g
Carbohydrates 82 g

Proteins 14 g

Ingredients

- 2 tablespoons olive oil
- 4 cloves garlic, finely chopped
- 1.5 pounds Arborio rice
- 6 tomatoes, chopped
- 2 teaspoons chopped rosemary
- 6 courgettes, finely diced
- 1 ¼ cups peas, fresh or frozen
- 12 cups hot vegetable stock
- 1 cup chopped
- Salt to taste
- Freshly ground pepper

CHILI CON CARNE

TIME **COOKING** **SERVE**
10 MINS 20 MINS 8

Method

1. Have your vegetables prepared. Chop into tiny dice 1 big onion, around 5 mm long. The best way to achieve so is to split the onion in half, peel it and then slice it lengthwise into a shape of thick matchsticks every second, not chopping them all to the root end because they are all kept together, round into dice over the match sticks.

2. Slice a red pepper in the half lengthwise, cut base, wash off the seeds, and then chop it. Then peel and cut 2 cloves of garlic.

3. Start off preparation. Place your pan over medium heat onto the hob. Apply 1 tbsp. of oil and keep on for 1 or 2 minutes before heated (if you use an electric hob a little longer).

4. Put the onion and cook for around 5 minutes, stirring relatively regularly, or until your onion is thick, squidgy and somewhat translucent.

5. Tip the 1 tsp. of hot chili powder or you can also add 1 tbsp. of soft chili powder, garlic, red pepper, and 1 tsp. of paprika then 1 tsp. of cumin ground.

6. Offer it a quick swirl, then leave for more 5 minutes to cook, stirring periodically.

7. Brown 500 g lean beef in a minced form, switch the flame up a little, add your meat to the saucepan and split it with the spatula or knife. When you insert the mince, the blend will sizzle a little bit.

Ingredients

- 1 tsp. hot chilli powder
- 1 tsp. paprika
- 1 large onion
- 2 tbsp. tomato purée
- 1 red pepper
- 1 tsp. ground cumin
- 1 tbsp. oil
- 1 beef stock cube
- 2 garlic cloves
- 1 tsp. sugar (you can also add a little piece of dark chocolate)
- 410g can red kidney beans
- 400g can chopped tomatoes
- 500g minced beef
- ½ tsp. dried marjoram
- Plain boiled long grain rice, to serve
- Soured cream, to serve

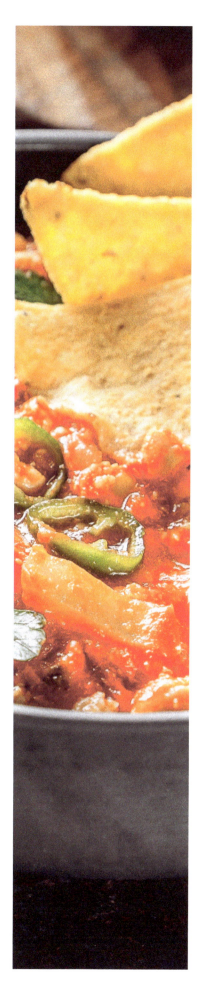

8. Keep mixing and prodding for 5 minutes at least, before all mince thing is in place, thin lumps and no pink parts are left. Keep your heat hot enough to fry the meat and turn brown, rather to just stewing.

9. Create a sauce. Crumble 1 cube of beef reserve into 300ml of hot broth. Pour it in the mixture being miNced into the pan.

10. Add chopped tomatoes to a 400 g bowl. Top with ½ tsp. of dried marjoram, 1 tsp. of sugar and then add a good pepper and salt shake. Sprinkle with some 2 tbsp. of tomato purée and then stir well the sauce.

11. Simmer softly around it. Bring the whole to the boil, stir well and put a cover on the saucepan. Shift the heat down until it spills softly, then quit for almost 20 minutes.

12. Occasionally check on the skillet to mix it, to be sure that the sauce does not stick on the bottom of the pan or dried out. If so, apply a couple tablespoons of water, and ensure that the heat is very small enough. The saucy, minced mixture should look moist, thick and juicy after gently simmering.

13. Drain and then rinse in a sieve a 410 g can of your kidney beans, then mix them into chili pot. Boil again, and bubble gently for more 10 minutes without the lid, you can add a little water more if it looks dry.

14. Taste a little of the season and chilli. Possibly, it would require far much seasoning than you thought.

15. Now remove the cover, turn off the flame and allow the chilli to remain until serving for about10 minutes. This is very important because it requires blending of the flavors.

16. Serve with simple boiled large grain rice and some soured cream.

Nutrition

Calories 403, Fats 4 g, Carbohydrates 90 g, Proteins 10 g

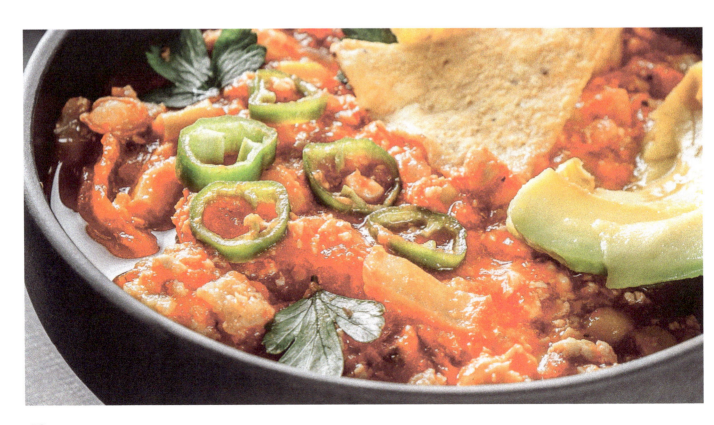

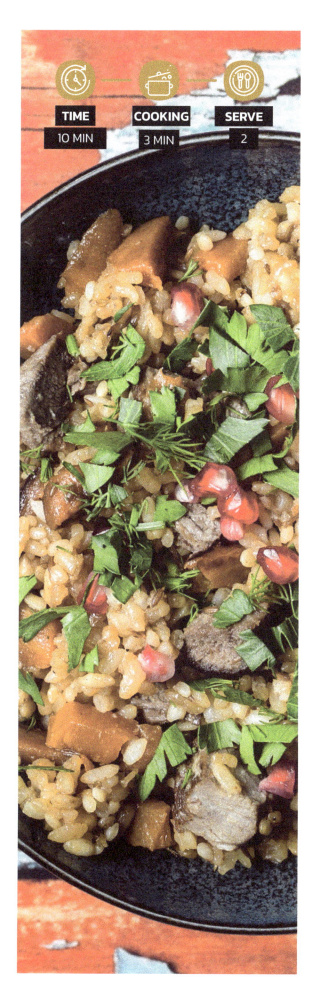

TIME 10 MIN | COOKING 3 MIN | SERVE 2

Brown Basmati Rice
PILAF

Ingredients

- ½ tablespoon vegan butter
- ½ cup mushrooms, chopped
- ½ cup brown basmati rice
- 2-3 tablespoons water
- 1/8 teaspoon dried thyme
- Ground pepper to taste
- ½ tablespoon olive oil
- ¼ cup green onion, chopped
- 1 cup vegetable broth
- ¼ teaspoon salt
- ¼ cup chopped, toasted pecans

Method

1. Place a saucepan over medium-low heat. Add butter and oil.

2. When it melts, add mushrooms and cook until slightly tender.

3. Stir in the green onion and brown rice. Cook for 3 minutes. Stir constantly.

4. Stir in the broth, water, salt and thyme.

5. When it begins to boil, lower heat and cover with a lid. Simmer until rice is cooked. Add more water or broth if required.

6. Stir in the pecans and pepper.

7. Serve.

Nutrition

Calories 189 Fats 11 g Carbohydrates 19 g Proteins 4 g

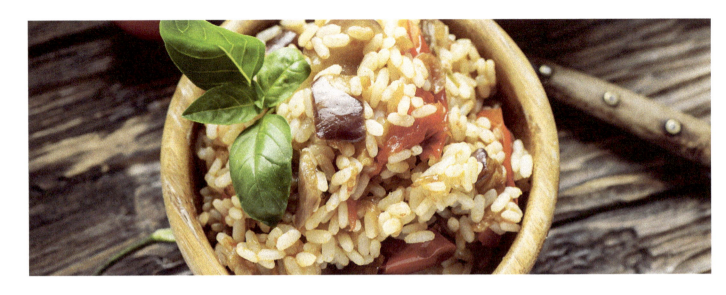

Artichoke & Eggplant
RICE

TIME 5 MINS **COOKING** 10 MINS **SERVE** 3

Method

1. Place a nonstick pan or paella pan over medium heat. Add 1 tablespoon oil. When the oil is heated, add eggplant and cook until brown all over.

2. Remove with a slotted spoon and place on a plate lined with paper towels.

3. Add 1 tablespoon oil. When the oil is heated, add onion and sauté until translucent.

4. Stir in garlic and parsley stalks. Cook for 10 minutes. Add all the spices and rice and stir-fry for a few minutes until rice is well coated with the oil.

5. Add salt and mix well. Pour half the broth and cook until dry. Stir occasionally.

6. Add eggplant and artichokes and stir. Pour remaining stock and cook until rice is tender. Add parsley leaves and lemon juice and stir.

7. Serve hot with lemon wedges.

Nutrition

Calories 431 Fats 16 g
Carbohydrates 58 g Proteins 8

Ingredients

- 2 tablespoons olive oil
- 1 medium onion, finely chopped
- A handful parsley, chopped
- 1 teaspoon turmeric powder
- 3 cups vegetable stock
- Juice, lemon
- 1 eggplant, chopped into chunks
- 1 clove garlic, crushed
- 1 teaspoon smoked paprika
- 7 ounces paella rice
- 1 package chargrilled artichoke
- Lemon wedges to serve

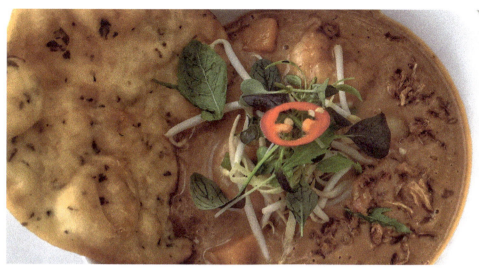
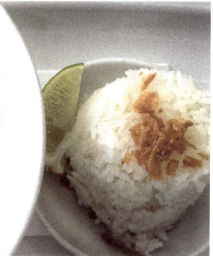

THAI RED CURRY

TIME
15 MINS

COOKING
60 MINS

SERVE
4

Ingredients

- 1 ½ cups packed thinly sliced kale
- Pinch of salt, more to taste
- 2 tablespoons Thai red curry paste
- 1 tablespoon soy sauce
- 1 ¼ cups long-grain brown jasmine rice
- 1 small white onion, chopped
- 1 tablespoon grated ginger
- 1 red bell pepper
- 1 tablespoon coconut oil or olive oil
- ½ cup water
- 1 ½ teaspoons of coconut sugar or turbinado sugar
- 2 cloves garlic
- 2 of teaspoons lime juice
- 3 carrots, peeled and sliced
- 1 bell pepper
- 1 can (14 ounces) regular coconut milk

Method

1. Take a big pot of water and put it to boil to prepare the rice. Insert the rinsed rice and start to boil for 30 minutes to avoid excess, decreasing heat when required. Remove from heat, drain rice, and put the rice back into the pot. Cover and let the rice rest until you are ready to serve for 10 minutes or longer. Season the rice to taste with salt just before serving, and fluff it with a fork.

2. To render the curry, fire up a broad skillet over medium fire with the deep sides, once warm, add your oil. Then add the onion and a sprinkle of salt and cook, stirring frequently for about 5 minutes until your onion has softened and turns translucent. Add the garlic and ginger, and cook for about 25-30 seconds while continuously stirring until fragrant.

3. Add the carrots and your bell peppers, cook, stirring regularly, until these bell peppers are fork-tender, 3 to 5 minutes more. Then add your curry paste, and cook for about 2 minutes, stirring frequently.

4. Add the water, kale, coconut milk, and sugar and whisk to mix. Bring in the mixture over medium flame to a simmer. Reduce flame as needed to keep a mild simmer and cook until the carrots, peppers, and kale have softened to your liking, stirring occasionally for about 5–10 minutes.

5. Remove your pot from flame and season with rice vinegar and tamari. Add salt (for optimum flavor), to taste. If your curry requires a little of more energy, add 1/2 teaspoon more tamari, or add 1/2 teaspoon more of your rice vinegar for more acidity. Divide both curry and rice into bowls and garnish them, if you like, with sliced cilantro and a sprinkle of your red pepper flakes. Serve on the side with sriracha or chili garlic sauce, if you like spicy curries.

6. If you want to add Tofu, first bake it and add it with coconut milk in step 4. If you apply raw tofu, it will take up so much of the fat, so baking it would enhance the flavor considerably, anyway.

Nutrition

Calories 133, Fats 15 g, Carbohydrates 17 g, Proteins 6 g

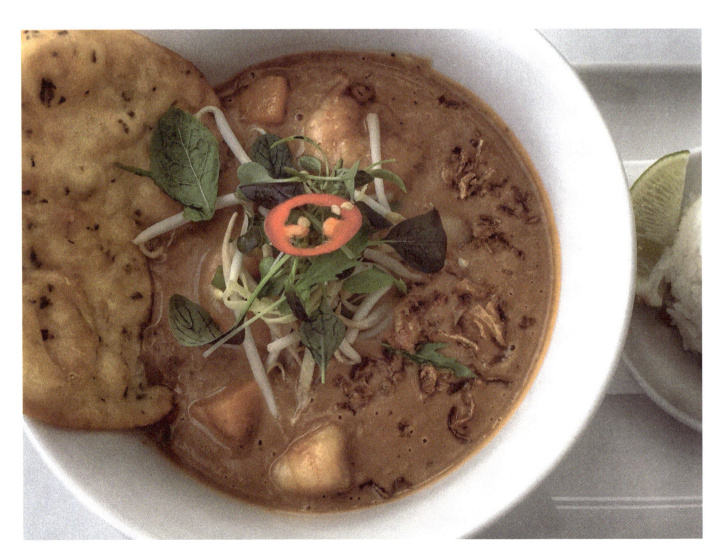

DESSERT RECIPES

PHASE 2

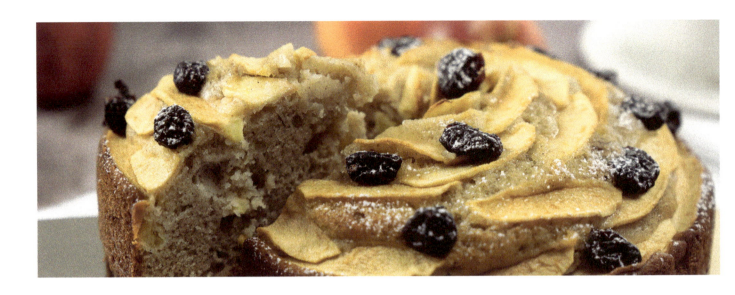

APPLE-RAISIN CAKE

TIME 15 MINS **COOKING** 50 MINS **SERVE** 12

Method

1. Spray an 8 x 8 x 2-inch baking pan with nonstick cooking spray and set aside. Into a medium bowl sift together flour, cinnamon, and cloves; set aside.

2. Preheat oven to 350°F. In a medium mixing bowl, using an electric mixer, cream margarine, add sugar and stir to combine. Stir baking soda into applesauce, then add to margarine mixture and stir to combine; add sifted ingredients and, using an electric mixer on medium speed, beat until thoroughly combined. Fold in apples and raisins; pour batter into the sprayed pan and bake for 45 to 50 minutes (until cake is browned and a cake tester or toothpick, inserted in center, comes out dry). Remove cake from pan and cool on wire rack.

3. This cake may be frozen for future use; to make serving easier, slice cake into individual portions, then wrap each portion in plastic freezer wrap and freeze. When ready to use, thaw the number of portions needed at room temperature.

Nutrition

Per serving 151 calories 2 g protein 4 g fat; 28 g carbohydrate 96 mg sodium; 0 mg cholesterol

Ingredients

- One teaspoon baking soda
- 1/2 cups applesauce (no sugar added)
- Two small Golden Delicious apples, cored, pared, and shredded
- 1 cup less 2 tablespoons raisins
- 2/4 cups self-rising flour
- 1 teaspoon ground cinnamon
- 1/2 teaspoon ground cloves 1/3 cup plus 2 teaspoons unsalted margarine
- 1/4 cup granulated sugar

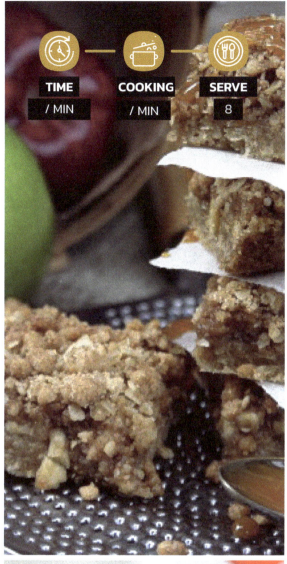

TIME / MIN COOKING / MIN SERVE 8

Apple-Nut
SQUARES

Ingredients

- 3/4 cup all-purpose flour
- 1 teaspoon double-acting baking powder
- 1 egg
- 2 tablespoons plus
- 2 teaspoons firmly packed dark brown sugar
- 1/2 cup chunky-style peanut butter
- 1 teaspoon vanilla extract
- 1/2 teaspoon ground cinnamon
- 1/4 cup skim milk
- 2 small Golden Delicious apples, cored, pared, and diced

Method

Preheat oven to 350°F. Onto sheet of wax paper or a paper plate sift together flour and baking powder; set aside. In a medium mixing bowl, combine egg and sugar and, using an electric mixer, beat until thick; add peanut butter, vanilla, and cinnamon and beat until combined. Add sifted flour alternately with milk, about V3 at a time, beating after each addition; stir in apple. Spray an 8 x 8 x 2-Inch baking pan with nonstick cooking spray; spread batter evenly in pan and bake until top is lightly browned, 30 to 35 minutes. Remove pan to wire rack and let cool for 5 minutes; remove the cake from pan and return to rack to cool completely. Cut into sixteen 2-inch squares.

Nutrition

184 calories 7 g protein 9 g fat 21 g carbohydrate

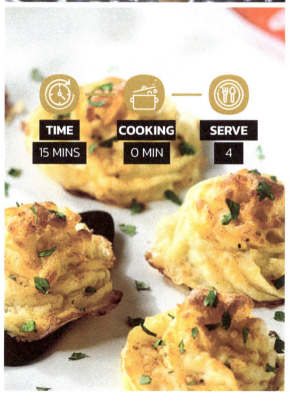

TIME 15 MINS COOKING 0 MIN SERVE 4

Potato
ROSETTES

Ingredients

- 8 ounces sliced pared potatoes, cooked and drained
- 2 tablespoons buttermilk
- 1 tablespoon plus 1 teaspoon each grated Parmesan cheese, divided, and margarine
- 1/2 teaspoons each minced fresh parsley and frozen or chopped fresh chives
- 1/4 teaspoon salt
- Dash white pepper

Method

1. Force potatoes through a food mill or coarse sieve into a 1-quart mixing bowl; add milk, 1 tablespoon cheese, and the margarine and seasonings and combine thoroughly.

2. Spray baking sheet with nonstick cooking spray.-Fit a pastry bag with a large rosette tube and fill the bag with potato mixture; pipe out mixture onto the sheet, forming 8 spiral

cones, each about 2 inches In diameter (if pastry bag is not available, spoon potato mixture onto the sprayed sheet, forming 8 mounds). Sprinkle each potato cone (or mound with 1/2 teaspoon cheese and broil, about 6 inches from the heat source, just until golden brown.

Nutrition

Per serving: 88 calories, 2 g protein, 4 g fat

Yogurt-Fruit PIE

TIME 15 MINS   **COOKING** 6 MINS   **SERVE** 8

Method

1. To Prepare Crust: Preheat oven to 350°F. Spray 9-inch glass pie plate with nonstick cooking spray; set aside.

2. In small bowl combine crumbs and margarine, mixing thoroughly; using the back of a spoon, press crumb mixture over bottom and up sides of sprayed pie plate. Bake until crust is crisp and brown, about 10 minutes; remove to wire rack and let cool.

3. To Prepare Filling: Pour orange juice into a small saucepan. Combine sugar and gelatin and sprinkle over juice; let stand for 1 minute to soften. Cook over medium-low heat, constantly stirring, until sugar and gelatin are completely dissolved; set aside.

4. In a medium bowl, using a wire whisk, gently stir together yogurt and pineapple; add gelatin mixture and vanilla and stir until thoroughly blended. Pour mixture into cooled pie crust; cover and refrigerate until firm, overnight or at least 4 hours.

5. To Serve: Arrange fruit decoratively over filling; serve immediately or cover and refrigerate until ready to use.

Nutrition

Per serving 202 calories 6 g protein 6 g fat 33 g carbohydrate

Ingredients

- Crust
- 16 graham crackers, made into crumbs
- 1/2 cup thawed frozen concentrated orange juice (no sugar added)
- 2 tablespoons plus 2 teaspoons granulated sugar
- 1 envelope unflavored gelatin
- Topping
- 40 small seedless green grapes
- 2 small nectarines, pitted and sliced
- 2 tablespoons plus 2 teaspoons margarine, softened
- 2 cups plain low-fat yogurt
- 1/2 cup canned crushed pineapple (no sugar added)
- 1 teaspoon vanilla extract
- 1/4 cup sliced strawberries

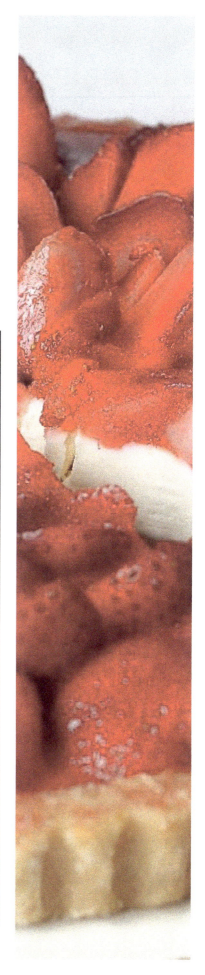

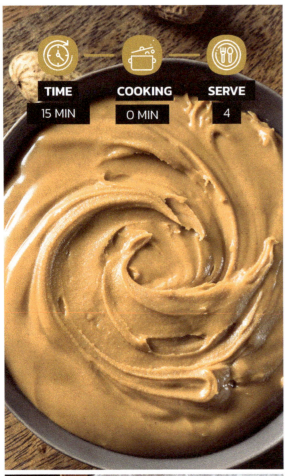

Creamy Peanut
DIP

Ingredients

- 1 tablespoon lemon juice
- 1/2 cup plain low-fat yogurt
- Dash vanilla extract
- 1/4 cup smooth peanut butter
- 3 tablespoons water
- 2 tablespoons thawed frozen concentrated orange juice (no sugar added)

Method

1. In a small bowl, combine peanut butter, water, and juices, mixing until smooth, stir in yogurt and vanilla. Cover and refrigerate until chilled.

2. Delicious served with fresh fruit (e.g., apples, pears, bananas, etc.) or carrot and celery sticks.

Nutrition

Per serving: 126 calories, 6 g protein, 8 g fat

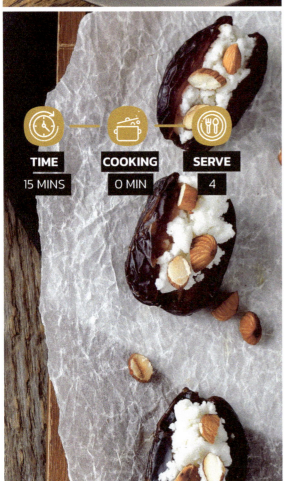

Stuffed
DATES

Ingredients

- 8 pitted dates, split open lengthwise
- 1/2 teaspoon confectioners' sugar
- 1/4 cup smooth peanut butter
- 2 teaspoons grated fresh orange peel, divided

Method

1. In a small bowl, combine peanut butter and 1 teaspoon orange peel; spoon 1/2 of the mixture into each date. Sift an equal amount of sugar over each filled date, then sprinkle each with 1/2 of the remaining orange peel.

Nutrition

Per serving: 141 calories, 5 g protein, 8 g fat, 16 g carbohydrate

OTHER RECIPES

PHASE 1 - part 1

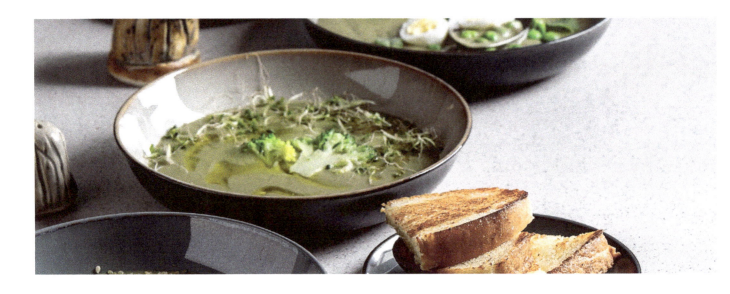

SOUP 'GREEN

TIME 15 MINS   **COOKING** 0 MINS   **SERVE** 1

Method

1. Wash and chop all the ingredients. Insert them into the glass of blender and crush.

2. Add the water and crush again until you get a homogeneous texture. If necessary, rectify water.

3. Take the soup as a snack at any time of the day to purify the body and keep cravings at bay. To know more: This cold soup is quick to prepare and has great benefits for the body. Perhaps the best-known property of the apple is its intestinal regulatory action. If we eat it raw and with skin, it is useful to treat constipation, since this way we take advantage of its richness in insoluble fiber present in the skin, which stimulates the intestinal activity and helps to keep the intestinal muscles in shape. Also, green apples are one of the largest sources of flavonoids. These antioxidant compounds can stop the action of free radicals on the cells of the body. Eating raw fruits and vegetables is the healthiest option.

Nutrition

Calories 330 Fat 12 g 18 % Cholesterol 90 mg Sodium 240 mg 10 % Carbohydrate 20 g 6 % Fiber 5 g 22 % Sugars 4 g Iron 15 %

Ingredients

- Water in sufficient quantity to achieve the desired texture
- 1 green apple with skin
- 1 slice of fresh peeled ginger
- Half lemon or 1 lime without skin, the white part without seeds
- Half cucumber with skin
- Half bowl of leaves with fresh spinach
- 1 bunch of basil or fresh cilantro
- 1 branch of wireless celery, including tender green leaves

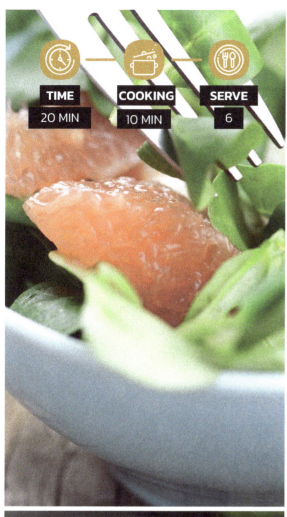

Pea Salad, Gourmet Peas, GRAPEFRUIT

TIME 20 MIN | **COOKING** 10 MIN | **SERVE** 6

Ingredients

- 1 pink grapefruit
- 800 g shelled peas
- 200 g gourmet peas
- 2 fresh onions with the stem
- 1 tray of sprouted seeds
- 1 drizzles of olive oil
- 1 dash of apple cider vinegar
- 1 tablespoon old-fashioned mustard
- Seeds sesame toasted

Method

1. Peel the grapefruit and collect the flesh (without the white skin), as well as the juice.

2. Steam peas 3-4 minutes and gourmet peas a little more

3. Mix the mustard in a salad bowl with the grapefruit juice, olive oil, vinegar, salt and pepper. Add the chopped onions with the stem, the vegetables and the grapefruit flesh. Mix well, sprinkle with sesame and sprinkle with sprouted seeds.

Nutrition

Calories: 1 Cal / Pers.

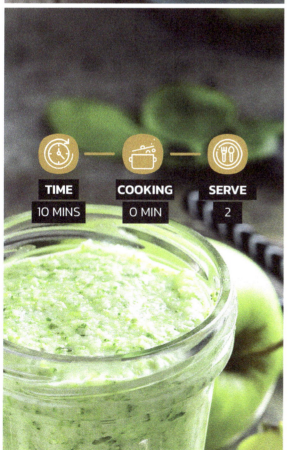

Detoxifying MILKSHAKE

TIME 10 MINS | **COOKING** 0 MIN | **SERVE** 2

Ingredients

- 1 cup of Celery (one head)
- 2 glass of Spinach
- 2 glass of Cucumber
- 1 unit (s) of Limón
- 2 unit (s) of Apple
- 1 pinch of fresh ginger

Method

1. Put the ingredients – Celery, Spinach, Cucumber, Limón, Apple, fresh ginger in the blender and then blend till a homogeneous mixture is obtained.

Nutrition

Composition Amount (gr) CDR (%) Calories 191.21 10% Carbohydrates 29.52 9.5% Proteins 7.32 15.3%

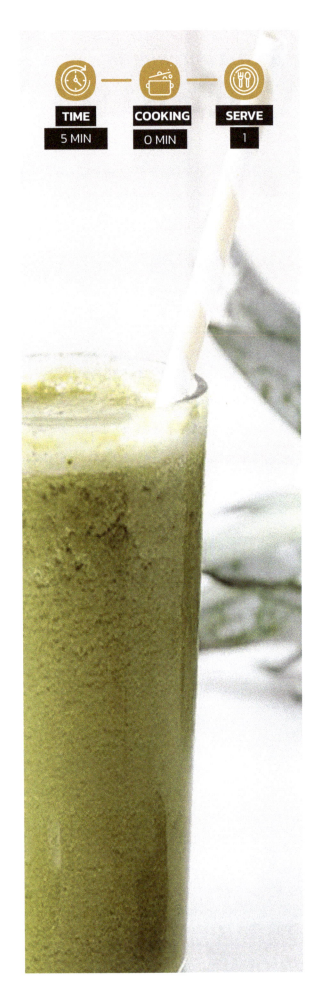

Green Pineapple
SMOOTHIE

Ingredients

- 50 grams of Chard
- 1 unit (s) of Apple
- 200 grams of Pineapple
- 1 teaspoon of Flax seeds

Method

1. Add Chard, Apple, Pineapple, Flax seeds all to the glass of the blender with a little water and grind well.

Nutrition

Calories 251.16 13.1% Carbohydrates 46.44 14.9% Proteins 3.51 7.3%

Cream of PEAR & ARAGULA

TIME 20 MINS **COOKING** 0 MINS **SERVE** 2

Method

1. Grind whole the ingredients in the blender jar, except extra virgin olive oil and flowers, until a creamy and homogeneous texture is obtained. If necessary, rectify water, salt, and pepper.

2. Refrigerate until ready to serve and, once in the bowl, decorate with the flowers and a thread of olive oil. If you do not have flowers, you can use chopped almonds, some rocket leaves or sesame seeds.

3. If you do not have a bowl of arugula you can also use other green leaves such as spinach, lamb's lettuce, watercress, mustard greens, etc. with the aromatic herbs, the same: you can make with parsley, dill, chives, basil, cilantro or mint. To know more: The pear is a fruit with satiating effect for its fiber content: it is fantastic for people who want to lose weight and are doing a diet to lose weight. Also, it is a fruit with anti-inflammatory action, helps us maintain a regular intestinal transit and combat constipation, and has a very beneficial effect on our micro biota or intestinal flora. Choose it whenever you can from organic farming.

Ingredients

- Half a liter of water
- 4 pears Banuelos with leather, at its point of maturation
- 1 bowl of arugula
- 2 tablespoons of fresh aromatic herbs
- The juice of 1 small lemon
- Sea salt or herbal salt
- 1 pinch of ground black pepper
- Extra virgin olive oil
- Edible flowers to decorate

Nutrition

Calories197.1 Total Fat12.1 g Saturated Fat3.2 g Polyunsaturated Fat3.5 g Monounsaturated Fat4.1 g Cholesterol10.0 mg Sodium181.2 mg Potassium149.7 mg Total Carbohydrate21.3 g Dietary Fiber3.0 g Sugars15.9 g Protein3.5 g

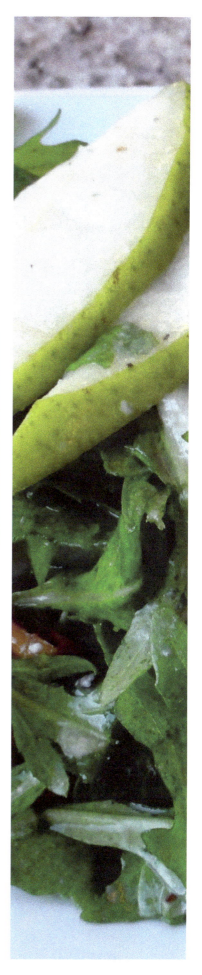

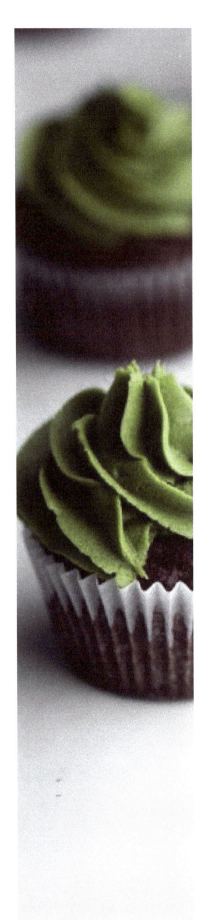

Chocolate Cupcakes with
MATCHA ICING -SIRT FOOD

TIME 10 MINS **COOKING** 20 MINS **SERVE** 12

Method

1. Preheat the stove to 180C/160C follower.

2. Place the flour, sugar, chocolate, salt and also espresso powder in a big bowl and mix thoroughly.

3. Include the milk, vanilla extract, vegetable oil and egg to the dry active ingredients and use an electric mixer to defeat until well-integrated. Very carefully pour in the boiling water slowly as well as beat on a low rate until completely incorporated. Make use of broadband to defeat for a more minute to include air to the batter. The batter is a lot more liquid than a regular cake mix. Have faith; it will certainly taste fantastic!

4. Spoon the batter uniformly in between the cake cases. Each cake instance ought to be no more than 3/4 full. Bake in the stove for 15-18 minutes, till the combination gets better when tapped. Remove from the oven and also enable to cool down entirely before icing.

5. To make the topping, lotion the butter and topping sugar together until it's pale and also smooth. Add the Matcha powder as well as vanilla and stir once again. Finally, add the lotion cheese as well as defeat up until smooth. Pipeline or topped the cakes.

Ingredients

- 150g self-rising flour
- 200g wheel sugar
- 60g cacao
- 1/2 tsp. salt
- 1/2 tsp. excellent espresso coffee, decaf if chosen
- 120ml milk
- 1/2 tsp. vanilla extract
- 50ml grease.
- One egg
- 120ml boiling water
- For the topping:
- 50g butter, at room temperature level.
- 50g topping sugar
- 1 tbsp. Matcha eco-friendly tea powder
- 1/2 tsp. vanilla bean paste
- 50g soft cream cheese

Nutrition

234 Cal

OTHER RECIPES

PHASE 1 - part 2

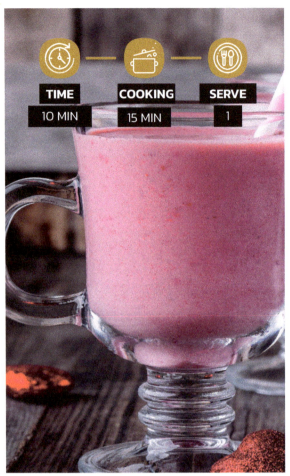

Creamy Strawberry & Cherry
SMOOTHIE

TIME 10 MIN | **COOKING** 15 MIN | **SERVE** 1

Ingredients

- 100g 3½ oz. strawberries
- 75g 3oz frozen pitted cherries
- 1 tablespoon plain full-fat yogurt
- 175mls 6fl oz. unsweetened soya milk

Method

1. Place the ingredients into a blender then process until smooth. Serve and enjoy.

Nutrition

132 calories per serving

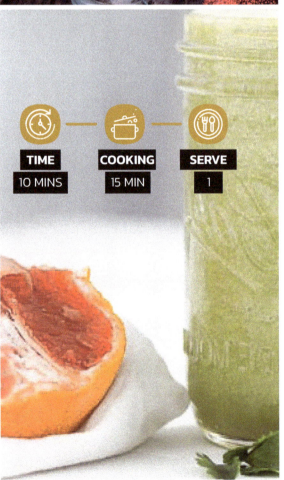

Grapefruit & Celery
BLAST

TIME 10 MINS | **COOKING** 15 MIN | **SERVE** 1

Ingredients

- 1 grapefruit, peeled
- 2 stalks of celery
- 50g 2oz kale
- ½ teaspoon Matcha powder

Method

1. Place ingredients into a blender with water to cover them and blitz until smooth.

Nutrition

71 calories per serving.

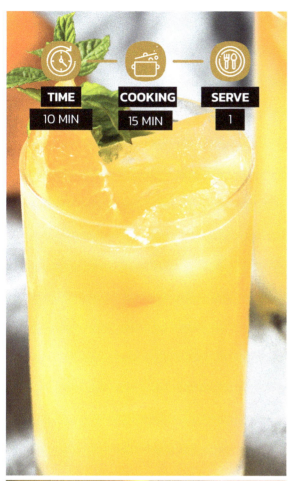

Orange & Celery
CRUSH

Ingredients
- 1 carrot, peeled
- 3 stalks of celery
- 1 orange, peeled
- ½ teaspoon Matcha powder
- Juice of 1 lime

Method
1. Place ingredients into a blender with enough water to cover them and blitz until smooth.

Nutrition
95 calories per serving.

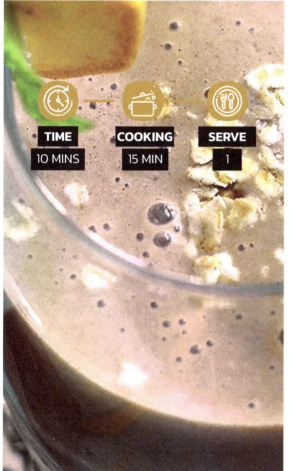

Tropical Chocolate
DELIGHT

Ingredients
- 1 mango, peeled & de-stoned
- 75g 3oz fresh pineapple, chopped
- 50g 2oz kale
- 25g 1oz rocket
- 1 tablespoon 100% cocoa powder or cacao nibs
- 150mls 5fl oz. coconut milk

Method
1. Place ingredients into a blender and blitz until smooth. You can add a little water if it seems too thick.

Nutrition
427 calories per serving.

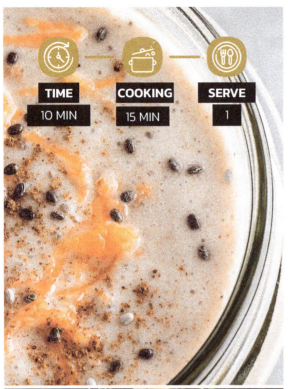

Walnut & Spiced Apple
TONIC

Ingredients

- 6 walnuts halves
- 1 apple, cored
- 1 banana
- ½ teaspoon Matcha powder
- ½ teaspoon cinnamon
- Pinch of ground nutmeg

Method

1. Place ingredients into a blender and add sufficient water to cover them, blitz until smooth and creamy

Nutrition

95 calories per serving.

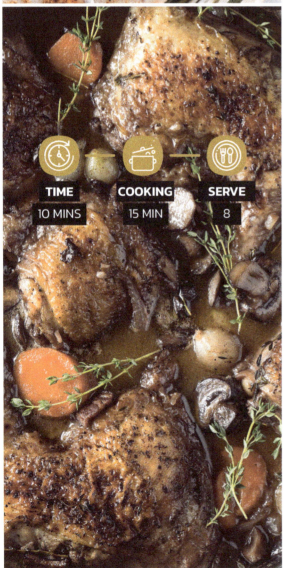

Coq Au
VIN

Ingredients

- 450g 1lb button mushrooms
- 100g 3½oz streaky bacon, chopped
- 16 chicken thighs, skin removed
- 3 cloves of garlic, crushed
- 3 tablespoons fresh parsley, chopped
- 3 carrots, chopped
- 2 red onions, chopped
- 2 tablespoons plain flour
- 2 tablespoons olive oil
- 750mls 1¼ pints red wine
- 1 bouquet grain

Method

1. In a large plate, put the flour and coat the chicken in it. Heat the olive oil then add the chicken and brown it, before setting aside. Fry the bacon in the pan then add the onion and cook for 5 minutes. Pour in the red wine and add the chicken, carrots, bouquet grain and garlic. Transfer it to a large ovenproof dish. Cook at 180C/360F for an hour. Remove the bouquet grain and skim off any excess fat, if necessary. Add in the mushrooms and cook for 15 minutes. Stir in the parsley just before serving.

Nutrition

459 calories per serving.

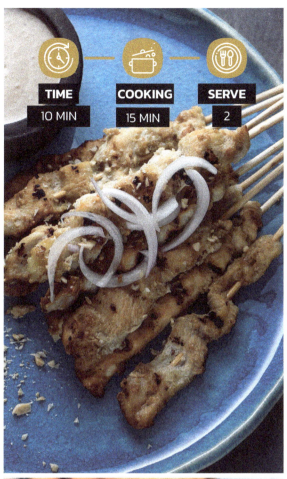

Turkey Satay
SKEWERS

TIME 10 MIN | **COOKING** 15 MIN | **SERVE** 2

Ingredients

- 250g 9oz turkey breast, cubed
- 25g 1oz smooth peanut butter
- 1 clove of garlic, crushed
- ½ small bird's eye chili or more if you like it hotter, finely chopped
- ½ teaspoon ground turmeric
- 200mls 7fl oz. coconut milk
- 2 teaspoons soy sauce

Method

1. Combine the coconut milk, peanut butter, turmeric, soy sauce, garlic and chili. Add the turkey pieces to the bowl and stir them until they are completely coated. Push the turkey onto metal skewers. Place the satay skewers on a barbeque or under a hot grill broiler and cook for 4-5 minutes on each side, until they are completely cooked.

Nutrition

431 calories per serving.

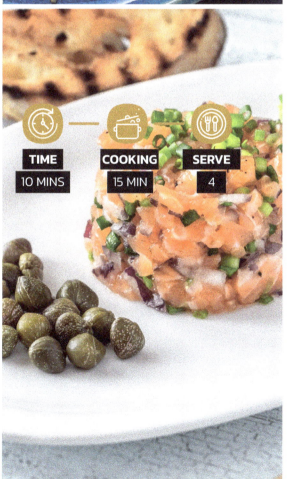

SALMON & CAPERS

TIME 10 MINS | **COOKING** 15 MIN | **SERVE** 4

Ingredients

- 75g 3oz Greek yogurt
- 4 salmon fillets, skin removed
- 4 teaspoons Dijon Mustard
- 1 tablespoon capers, chopped
- 2 teaspoons fresh parsley
- Zest of 1 lemon

Method

1. Put the yogurt, mustard, lemon zest, parsley and capers in a mixing bowl. Thoroughly coat the salmon in the mixture. Place the salmon under a hot grill broiler and cook for 3-4 minutes on each side, or until the fish is cooked. Serve with mashed potatoes and vegetables or a large green leafy salad.

Nutrition

321 calories per serving.

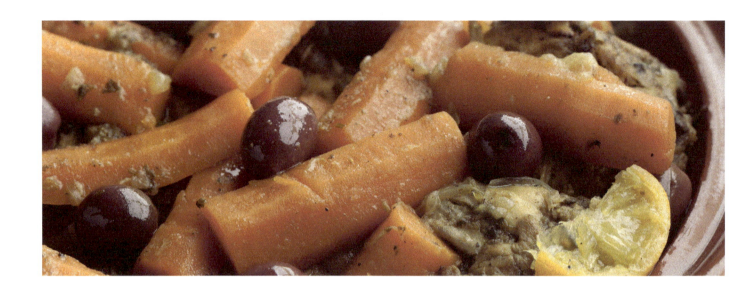

MOROCCAN CHICKEN CASSEROLE

TIME 10 MINS   **COOKING** 15 MINS   **SERVE** 4

Method

1. Place the chicken, chickpeas garbanzo beans, onion, carrot, chili, cumin, turmeric, cinnamon and stock broth into a large saucepan. Put it to the boil, and reduce heat after that simmer for 25 minutes. Add in the dates and apricots and simmer for 10 minutes. In a cup, mix the corn flour together with the water until it becomes a smooth paste. Pour the mixture into the saucepan and stir until it thickens. Add in the coriander cilantro and mix well. Serve with buckwheat or couscous.

Nutrition

401 calories per serving.

Ingredients

- 250g 9oz tinned chickpeas garbanzo beans drained
- 4 chicken breasts, cubed
- 4 Medrol dates, halved
- 6 dried apricots, halved
- 1 red onion, sliced
- 1 carrot, chopped
- 1 teaspoon ground cumin
- 1 teaspoon ground cinnamon
- 1 teaspoon ground turmeric
- 1 bird's-eye chili, chopped
- 600mls 1 pint's chicken stock broth
- 25g 1oz corn flour
- 60mls 2fl oz. water
- 2 tablespoons fresh coriander

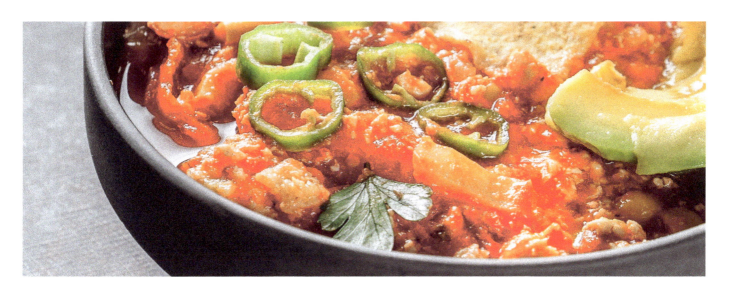

CHILI CON CARNE

TIME
10 MINS

COOKING
15 MINS

SERVE
4

Method

1. Put the oil in a saucepan then add the onion and cook for 5 minutes. Add in the garlic, celery, chili, turmeric, and cumin and cook for 2 minutes before adding then meat then cook for another 5 minutes. Pour in the stock broth, red wine, tomatoes, tomato purée, red pepper bell pepper, kidney beans and cocoa powder. Let it simmer for 45 minutes, keep it covered and stirring occasionally. Serve with brown rice or buckwheat.

Nutrition

390 calories per serving.

Ingredients

- 450g 1lb lean minced beef
- 400g 14oz chopped tomatoes
- 200g 7oz red kidney beans
- 2 tablespoons tomato purée
- 2 cloves of garlic, crushed
- 2 red onions, chopped
- 2 bird's-eye chilies, finely chopped
- 1 red pepper bell pepper, chopped
- 1 stick of celery, finely chopped
- 1 tablespoon cumin
- 1 tablespoon turmeric
- 1 tablespoon cocoa powder
- 400mls 14 FL oz. beef stock broth
- 175mls 6fl oz. red wine
- 1 tablespoon olive oil

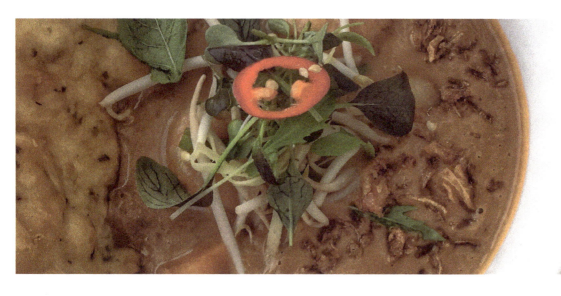
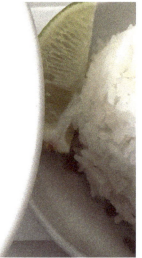

PRAWN & COCONUT CURRY

TIME
10 MINS

COOKING
15 MINS

SERVE
4

Method

1. Place the onions, garlic, tomatoes, chilies, lime juice, turmeric, ground coriander, chilies and half of the fresh coriander cilantro into a blender and blitz until you have a smooth curry paste. In a frying pan, put the oil, add the paste and cook for 2 minutes. Stir in the coconut milk and warm it thoroughly. Add the prawn's shrimps to the paste and cook them until they have turned pink and are completely cooked. Stir in the fresh coriander cilantro. Serve with rice.

Nutrition

322 calories per serving.

Ingredients

- 400g 14oz tinned chopped tomatoes
- 400g 14oz large prawns' shrimps, shelled and raw
- 25g 1oz fresh coriander cilantro chopped
- 3 red onions, finely chopped
- 3 cloves of garlic, crushed
- 2 bird's eye chilies
- ½ teaspoon ground coriander cilantro
- ½ teaspoon turmeric
- 400mls 14fl oz. coconut milk
- 1 tablespoons olive oil
- Juice of 1 lime

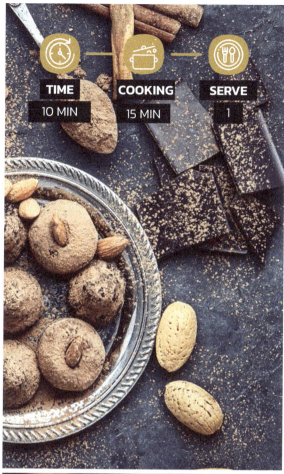

Choc Nut TRUFFLES

TIME 10 MIN | **COOKING** 15 MIN | **SERVE** 1

Ingredients

- 150g 5oz desiccated shredded coconut
- 50g 2oz walnuts, chopped
- 25g 1oz hazelnuts, chopped
- 4 Medrol dates
- 2 tablespoons 100% cocoa powder or cacao nibs
- 1 tablespoon coconut oil

Method

1. Place ingredients into a blender and process until smooth and creamy. Using a teaspoon, scoop the mixture into bite-size pieces then roll it into balls. Place them into small paper cases, cover them and chill for 1 hour before serving.

Nutrition

236 calories per serving.

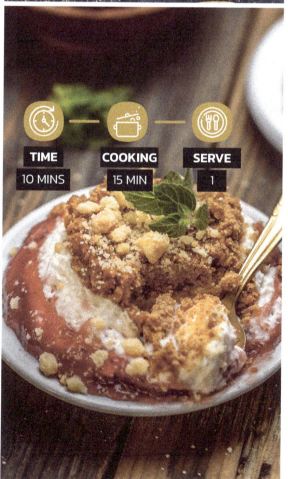

No-Bake Strawberry FLAPJACKS

TIME 10 MINS | **COOKING** 15 MIN | **SERVE** 1

Ingredients

- 75g 3oz porridge oats
- 125g 4oz dates
- 50g 2oz strawberries
- 50g 2oz peanuts unsalted
- 50g 2oz walnuts
- 1 tablespoon coconut oil
- 2 tablespoons 100% cocoa powder or cacao nibs

Method

1. Place ingredients into a blender and process until they become a soft consistency. Spread the mixture onto a baking sheet or small flat tin. Press the mixture down and smooth it out. Cut it into 8 pieces, ready to serve. You can add an extra sprinkling of cocoa powder to garnish if you wish.

Nutrition

182 calories each.

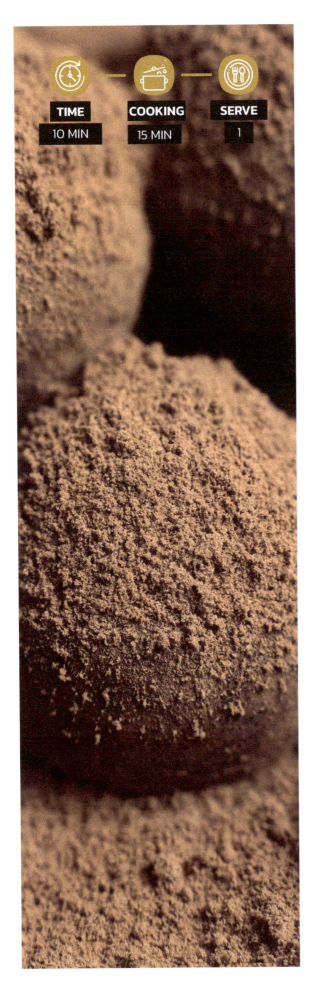

CHOCOLATE BALLS

TIME 10 MIN
COOKING 15 MIN
SERVE 1

Ingredients

- 50g 2oz peanut butter or almond butter
- 25g 1oz cocoa powder
- 25g 1oz desiccated shredded coconut
- 1 tablespoon honey
- 1 tablespoon cocoa powder for coating

Method

1. Mix all ingredients into a bowl. Scoop out a little of the mixture and shape it into a ball. Roll the ball in a little cocoa powder and set aside. Repeat for the remaining mixture. Can be eaten straight away or stored in the fridge.

Nutrition

115 calories per serving.

CHAPTER 2

FISH

Savory
SIRTFOOD SALMON

Method

Preheat your oven to 200 °C. Fry the celery, chili, garlic, onion, and ginger on olive oil up to three minutes. Add quinoa, tomatoes, and the chicken stock and let simmer for another ten minutes.

Layer olive oil, lemon juice, and turmeric on top of the salmon and bake for ten minutes. Add parsley and celery before serving.

Ingredients

- Salmon, 5 oz
- Lemon juice, 1 tbsp
- Ground turmeric, 1 tsp
- Extra virgin olive oil, 2 tbsp
- 1 chopped red onion
- 1 finely chopped garlic clove
- 1 finely chopped bird's eye chili
- Quinoa, 2 oz
- Finely chopped ginger, fresh, 1 tsp
- Celery, chopped, 1 cup
- Parsley, chopped, 1 tbsp
- Tomato, diced, 4.5 oz
- Vegetable stock, 100 ml

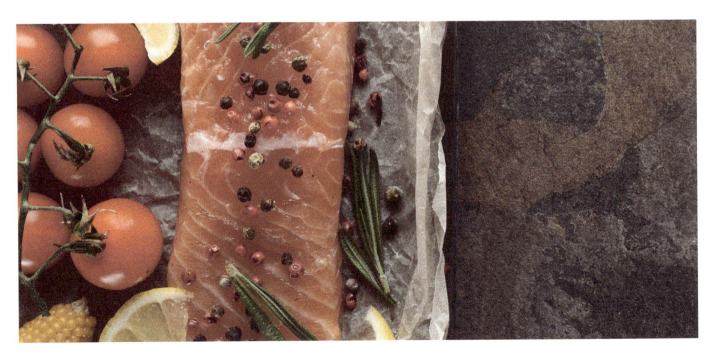

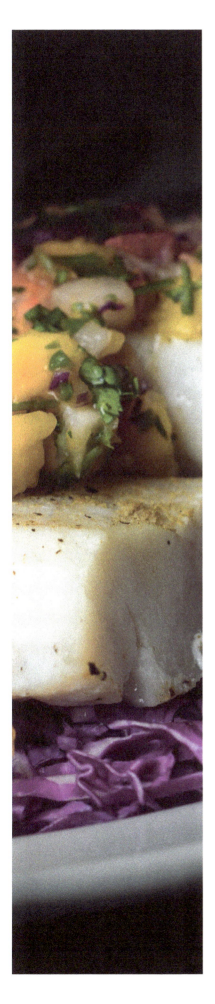

Fish with
MANGO & TUMERIC

Method

1. Marinate the fish and leave overnight

2. Blend the ingredients for mango dipping sauce

3. Fry the fish in 2 tbsp in coconut oil on medium heat and add a pinch of salt after five minutes. Turn to the other side and fry for another couple of minutes. Keep the remaining oil in the pan. Add scallions and dill and turn off the heat. Heat for about 15 seconds and season with a pinch of salt.

4. Top the fish with the infused oil, dill, and scallion and serve with the mango sauce, nuts, lime, and cilantro.

Ingredients

- A fresh 1 ¼ lbs piece of fish of your choosing
- ½ cup of coconut oil
- A pinch of sea salt
- 1 tbsp of high-quality red wine
- ¼ cup olive oil
- ½ tbsp minced ginger
- Scallion, 2 cup
- Dill, 2 cup
- 1 ripe mango
- 1 squeezed lemon
- 1 garlic clove
- Dry red pepper, 1 tsp
- Fresh cilantro
- Walnuts

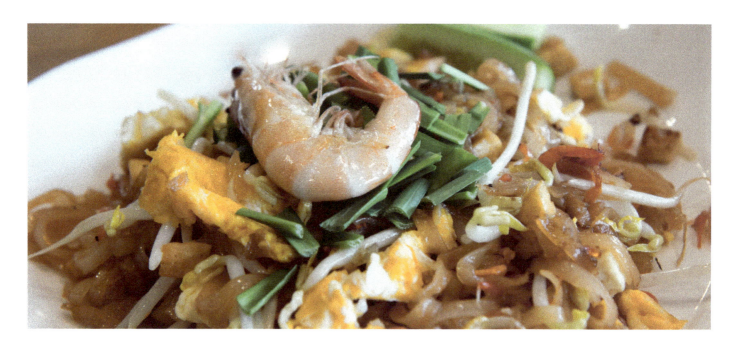

SIRTFOOD SHRIMP NOODLES

Method

Cook the shrimps in 1 tsp of the soy sauce and one tsp of the oil up to three minutes on high heat.

Cook buckwheat noodles for up to eight minutes and drain.

Fry the remaining ingredients in a pan on medium heat for up to three minutes. Add the chicken stock, bring to a boil, and cook until the veggies are cooked, but still look fresh. Add the shrimps and noodles, bring to a boil, and you're done!

Ingredients

- Shrimps, deveined ⅓ lb
- Soy sauce, 2 tsp
- Extra virgin olive oil, 2 tsp
- Buckwheat noodles, 3oz
- 2 finely chopped garlic cloves
- 1 bird's eye chili, finely chopped
- Chopped fresh ginger, 1 tsp
- Chopped red onion, ¼
- Chopped celery with eaves, ½ cup
- Chopped green beans, ½ cup
- Chopped kale, 1 cup
- Chicken stock, ½ cup

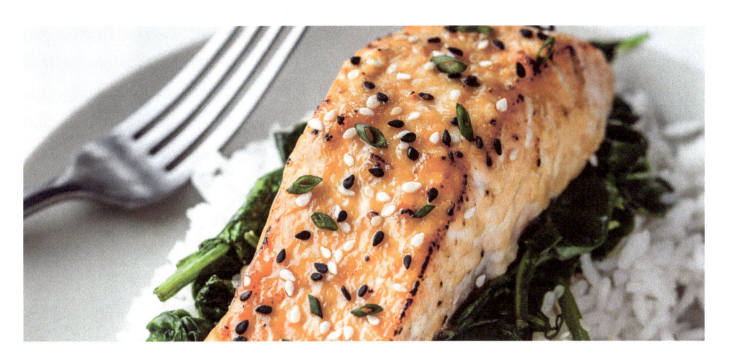

SIRTFOOD MISO SALMON

Method

1. Marinate the salmon in the mix of red wine, 1 tsp of extra virgin olive oil, and miso for 30 minutes. Preheat your oven to 420 °F and bake the fish for ten minutes.

2. Fry the onions, chili, garlic, green beans, ginger, kale, and celery for a few minutes until it's cooked. Insert the soy sauce, parsley, and sesame seeds.

3. Cook buckwheat per instructions and mix in with the stir-fry. Enjoy!

Ingredients

- Miso, ½ cup
- Organic red wine, 1 tbsp
- Extra virgin olive oil, 1 tbsp
- Salmon, 7 oz
- 1 sliced red onion
- Celery, sliced, 1 cup
- 2 finely chopped garlic cloves
- 1 finely chopped bird's eye chili
- Ground turmeric, 1 tsp
- Freshly chopped ginger, 1 tsp
- Green beans, 1 cup
- Kale, finely chopped, 1 cup
- Sesame seeds. 1 tsp
- Soy sauce, 1 tbsp
- Buckwheat, 2 tbsp

SIRTFOOD SALMON WITH KALE SALAD

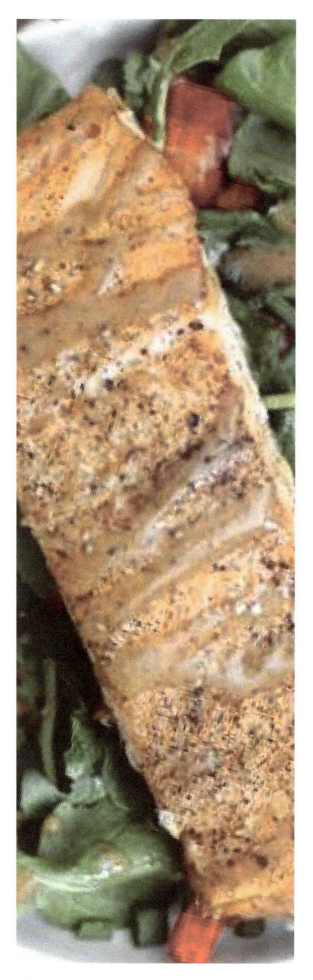

Ingredients

- Salmon, 4 oz
- 2 sliced red onions
- Parsley, chopped, 1 oz
- Cucumber, 2 oz
- 2 sliced radishes
- Spinach, ½ cup
- Salad leaves, ½ cup
- Salad dressing
- Raw honey, 1 tsp
- Greek yogurt, 1 tbsp
- Lemon juice, 1 tbsp
- Chopped mint leaves, 2 tbsp
- A pinch of salt
- A pinch of pepper

Method

1. Preheat your oven to 200 °C. Bake the salmon for up to 18 minutes and set aside. Mix in the ingredients for dressing and leave to sit between five and ten minutes.

2. Serve the salad with spinach and top with parsley, onions, cucumber, and radishes.

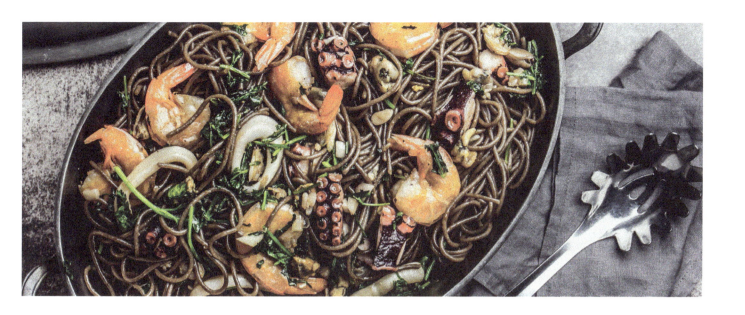

SIRTFOOD SHRIMPS WITH BUCKWHEAT NOODLES

Method

1. Cook the shrimps for three minutes on high heat and with 1 tsp of tamari and 1 tsp of extra virgin olive oil. Set aside.

2. Cook the noodles for up to eight minutes and set aside.

3. Fry kale, beans, celery, and onion, ginger, chili, and garlic in oil for up to three minutes. Add vegetable stock and simmer for two minutes.

4. Mix all together, bring to a boil, and serve.

Ingredients

- Shrimps (or a piece of fish of your choosing), 4 oz
- Tamari, 2 tbsp
- Extra virgin olive oil, 2 tbsp
- Buckwheat noodles, 75 g
- 1 finely chopped bird's eye chili
- 1 finely chopped garlic clove
- Fresh ginger, chopped, 1 tsp
- 1 sliced red onion
- Sliced red celery, ½ cup
- Chopped green beans, 1 cup
- Chopped kale, 1 cup
- Chicken stock, 1 cup
- Celery, 1 tsp

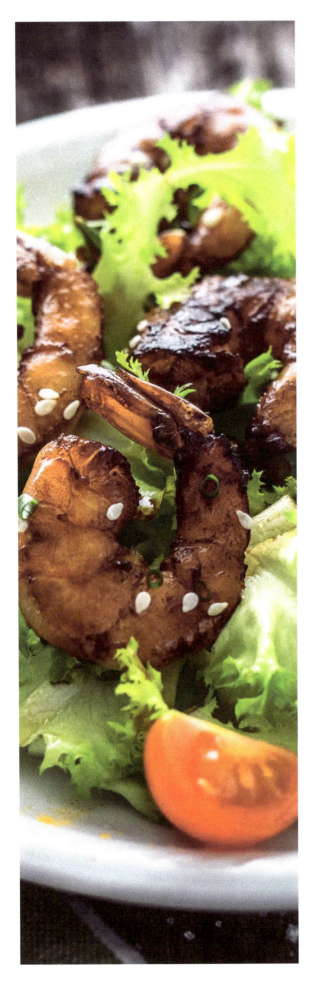

SIRTFOOD SHELLFISH SALAD

Ingredients

- Tomato sauce, 1 tsp
- Cloves, ¼ tsp
- Coriander, chopped, 1 tbsp
- Parsley, chopped, 1 tbsp
- Lemon juice, 1 tbsp (½ of a lemon)
- Kale, chopped, 1 cup
- Spinach, chopped, 1 cup
- Sea fruit of your choosing (shrimps, prawns, or clamps), 1 cup
- Chopped firm tofu, 1 thick slice (approx. 4 oz)
- Buckwheat noodles, 1 cup
- Pecan nuts, ½ cup
- Chopped ginger, ½ cup
- Miso paste, 1 tbsp
- Carrots, ½ cup
- Chicken stock, 100 ml

Method

Simmer tomato sauce with lemon juice, chicken stock, coriander, parsley, and shrimps/cloves/clams for 10 minutes on medium heat. Add the remaining ingredients without the ginger and miso, and stir-fry until the shellfish is cooked through. Add the remaining seasonings, and you're done !

SIRTFOOD PIZZA

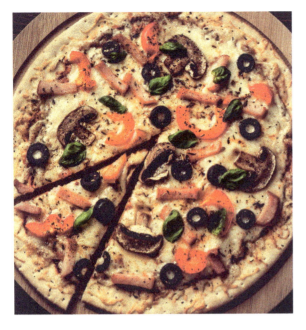

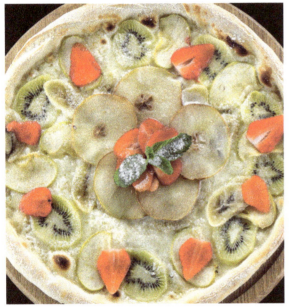

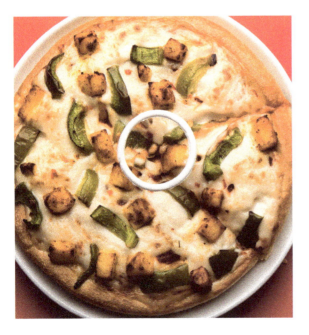

Sirtfood Pizzas are delicious and satiating, aside from being low-carb, low-calorie, and nutrient-rich. While you don't have to bake entirely Sirtfood pizzas to follow this diet plan, and instead you can just add individual Sirt foods to your favorite pizza, these recipes will fit into your 1,000–1,500 daily calorie limit. Here's how to bake two small Sirtfood pizzas:

Method

1. Start off by making the dough. First, dissolve the yeast in water and add sugar. Leave up to 15 minutes covered in clingfilm.

2. Next, slowly pour the flour into the bowl. Pay attention not to create clumps as you pour the flour into the yeast.

3. Add the extra virgin olive oil and start mixing the dough. Proceed to knead until the mix is smooth, consistent, and thick.

4. Leave the dough to rise up to 60 minutes in an oiled bowl, after you've covered it with a damp cloth or a tea towel. You'll know the dough has risen enough when it doubles in size.

5. While your dough rises, start making your sauce. Start by frying chopped garlic and onion in a small dose of olive oil. Once the onion softens, pour in the wine and add dried oregano. Proceed cooking until the mixture reduces by half.

6. Add chopped tomatoes, stir, and pour the sugar into the sauce. Proceed cooking for another 30 minutes. Wait until your dough rises and knead for a couple more minutes to remove the air bubbles. Heat your oven to 220 °C. Dust your kitchen counter with flour, split the dough into halves, and roll out the pieces until you like their thickness. Transfer onto the baking tray or the pizza stone.

7. Now layer the tomato sauce over the dough and leave a small gap along the edges. Add the toppings you like, and in quan-

tities you prefer. However, make sure to add any heat sensitive ingredients, like arugula or chili, after you've baked the pizza. Leave for another 15 minutes for the dough to start rising again. Bake for up to 12 minutes. Once your pizza is out of the oven, add fresh herbs and toppings of your choosing.

Ingredients

- Base
- Flour, 14 oz (½ buckwheat flour, ½ rice or white flour)
- Water, 3 cup
- 1 bag of dried yeast
- 1 tbsp of extra virgin olive oil
- 1 tsp of brown sugar
- Sauce
- 14 oz of chopped tomatoes, fresh or canned
- ½ chopped red onion
- 1 chopped garlic clove
- 2 tbsp of red wine
- 1 tsp of extra virgin olive oil
- Dried oregano, 1 tsp
- Basil leaves, 1 tsp
- Toppings
- Grilled eggplant, red onion, arugula
- Cherry tomato, chili flakes, cottage cheese or mozzarella
- Olives, cooked chicken
- Kale (fresh and steamed), chorizo, mushrooms, red onions

Great job! *You now know which meals to cook during your Sirtfood diet calorie restriction. Rest assured that these recipes will help you feel full and energized throughout the entire day. Here are some general tips and tricks for more convenient Sirtfood cooking:*

- *Be practical. Most of the recipes given in this chapter won't take longer than 30-45 minutes to make. However, you can make the process even faster and easier by pre-making meals the day or night before, or cooking larger amounts of meat and vegetables and storing your meals in the fridge.*
- *Invest in quality pots. Quality cooking supplies guarantee that you'll be able to stir-fry without using a lot of oil. The majority of recipes given in this chapter are easy to cook*

with no more than 2 tbsp of extra virgin olive oil. But, without the right dishes, it could happen that your foods start to stick to the bottom of the pan. In this case, instead of adding more oil, simply pour a little bit of water.

- *Substitutes. Don't like some of the ingredients provided in these recipes? Or, you find some of them difficult to find or expensive to purchase? Don't worry! Each of these meals can be adjusted according to your taste. Here are a couple of substitutes that you can use for some of the ingredients:*

1. **Meat**. *You can substitute different types of meat for an equal amount of any other meat you like. You can also substitute meat with mushrooms, potatoes, eggs, and beans.*
2. **Fruit**. *If you don't want to use avocados, you can replace them with bananas or melons. Melons have a similar consistency, and while they don't taste the same as avocados, they won't significantly alter a dish.*
3. **Buckwheat**. *As you may have noticed, buckwheat is heavily featured in the majority of recipes. If you don't want to eat that much of it, you can switch it with an equal amount of quinoa, kale, spinach, or beans. Keep in mind that doing so will affect the steps in cooking, and may affect preparation time. If you're not using leafy greens to substitute buckwheat, but you're using beans or legumes instead, it would be the best to cook the substitutes beforehand, and add them to other dishes as they're being cooked.*

CHAPTER 4

VEGETARIAN SIRTFOOD RECIPES

You can follow the Sirtfood diet even if you're a vegetarian or a vegan. The 20 superfoods and the diet principles that aim to trigger your 'skinny' gene don't include any animal ingredients, meaning that you can have all the Sirt foods you want and in abundant amounts. Aside from that, this diet doesn't exclude any plant-based foods from your daily meal plan, meaning that you most likely won't have to give up your favorite go-to meals throughout the diet.

However, due to the calorie restrictions in the first two phases of the diet, you should give your nutrition some extra attention and even use supplements if needed to make sure you're covered with the essential nutrients. Compared to the carnivore diet, calorie restriction during the first two weeks can feel extra hard, because you might be deprived of the nutrients otherwise found in meat and dairy, like protein. To secure healthy nutrition during the diet, you should supplement iodine, calcium, omega-3 fatty acids, and vitamin B12.

Sirt foods are compatible with any other diet approach you might be following, and don't require you to eliminate any food groups. The only restrictive element of the diet revolves around calories. During the first week, even as a vegetarian, your calorie count will total 1,000 calories, and you should aim for 1,500 calories during your second week. With this in mind, you should still aim to design your meals so that 50% of your serving consists of healthy, organic carbs, 25% fiber (fruits and vegetables), and 25% protein (meats or protein-dense plants). Taking this into consideration, you should aim to have 750 calories-worth of carbs, 350 calories from fiber, and 350 calories from protein-based foods. While there's no secure way to ensure your proportions are accurate, getting as close to these numbers will give your body all the nutrition it needs to function properly, despite the calorie restriction. Research showed that even people with chronic illnesses felt well and improved not only their weight but also blood sugar and blood pressure when their diet was balanced. Numerous studies recorded similar results even when participants with obesity were put on highly restrictive, 1000-calorie daily diets, and even when they fasted for longer periods. This only goes to show that calorie restriction doesn't have to be difficult if you balance out your meals.

Keeping in mind that healthy carbs do provide an immediate energy source for you to feel good while your body burns fat, you can turn to starchy Sirt foods (soy, onions, kale, and buckwheat) and make them as abundant in your portions as possible while sticking to the maximum daily intake recommendations.

Aside from vegan and vegetarian, the Sirtfood diet is also compatible with gluten-free, low-carb, paleo, ketogenic, and intermittent fasting diet. If your diet is low-carb, and you feel like you're not having enough fruits and vegetables, which is all too common for the majority of people who don't have the time to study and plan their diets, the Sirtfood diet can be a really simple way to enhance your diet without additional calories. With a simple list of foods needed to reap the health benefits, you won't have a problem incorporating these foods without compromising your diet concept.

BREAKFAST

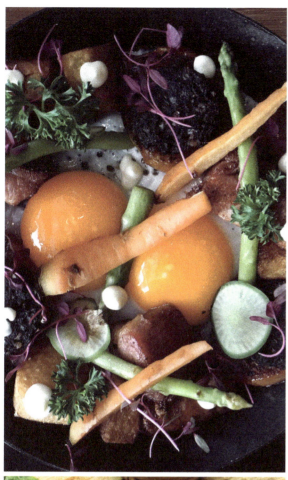

Eggs and Sirtfood VEGETABLES

Ingredients

- 1 eggs
- Kale, chopped, 1 cup
- Chopped parsley, 1 tbsp
- Chopped red onion, ½ cup
- Extra virgin olive oil, 1 tsp
- 1 finely chopped garlic clove
- Finely chopped celery, ½ cup
- 1 finely chopped paprika or bird's eye chili
- Ground turmeric, 1 tsp
- Ground cumin, 1 tsp
- Paprika, 1 tsp, 1 14 oz can of sliced tomatoes

Method

Fry the chili, spices, garlic, onion, and celery for a minute or two in olive oil, add the tomato sauce and let it simmer for 20 minutes. Pop the kale into the pan and cook for another five minutes, adding more water as needed. Lastly, add the parsley. Break the eggs and stir into the sauce, or boil them and serve next to the sauce.

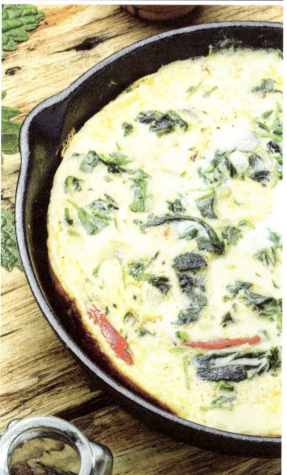

Vegetarian Sirtfood OMELET

Ingredients

- 2 eggs
- Kale, chopped, ½ cup
- Ground turmeric, 1 tsp
- Ginger, finely chopped, 1 tsp
- 1 sliced bird's eye chili
- Extra virgin olive oil, 1 tsp

Method

Mix all ingredients together. Optionally, you can blend for a minute if you prefer a homogenous-looking omelet. Fry in olive oil. First, layer the eggs across the frying pan and wait for the edges to turn dry and golden. Flip and fry on the other side.

Sirtfood Fruit YOGURT

Ingredients

- Strawberries, chopped, 1 cup
- Raspberries, 1 cup
- Greek yogurt, 2 cup
- Chia seeds, 1 tbsp

Method

Blend the berries with Greek yogurt and chia seeds and enjoy!

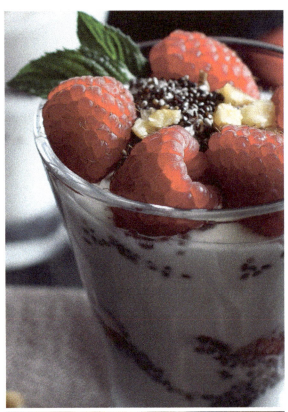

Buckwheat Apple PANCAKES

This recipe will give your four quick, healthy, and delicious pancakes.

Ingredients

- Two eggs
- Buckwheat flour, 2 cup
- Sugar, 2 tbsp
- A pinch of salt
- Two chopped, peeled apples
- Skim milk, 3 cup
- Olive oil, 2 tsp
- Baking powder, 1 tsp

Method

1. Cook apples in a small amount of water, up to ½ cup and let boil up to two minutes. Blend to create a sauce.

2. Now, start making pancakes. Mix baking powder, the flour, and sugar into a bowl. Add milk and mix until the texture is even and smooth. Mix in both eggs.

3. Fry ¼ of the batter on ½ tsp of olive oil on medium high heat. Repeat four times, until you fry all of the batter.

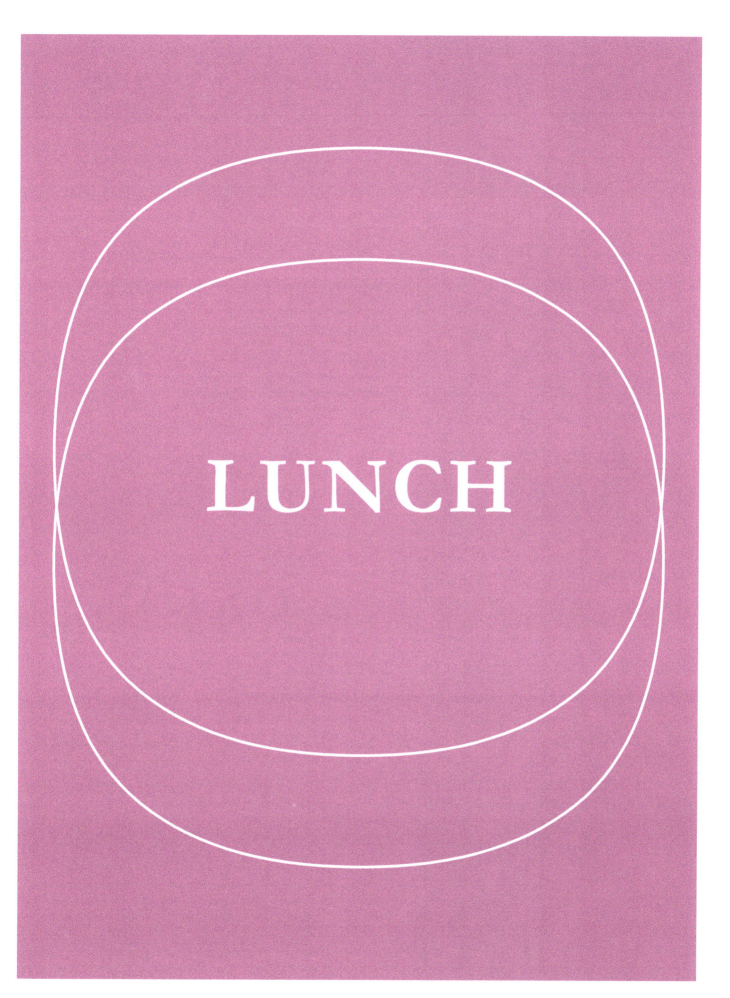

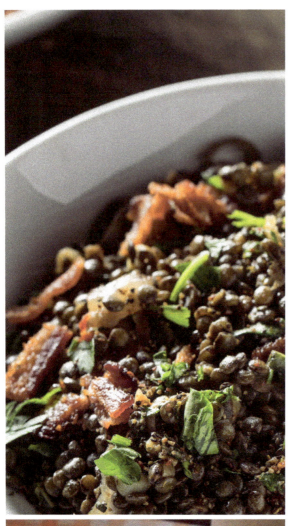

Sirtfood LENTILS

Ingredients

- 1 cup chopped cherry tomatoes
- Extra virgin olive oil, 2 tsp
- 1 finely chopped red onion
- 1 finely chopped garlic clove
- Celery, thin-sliced, ½ cup
- Carrots, diced, ½ cup
- Paprika or bird's eye chili, 1 tsp
- Thyme, dry or fresh, 1 tsp
- Parsley, 1 tbsp, Arugula, 20 g
- Chopped kale, 1 cup
- Lentils, 1 cup, Vegetable stock, 220 ml

Method

Preheat your oven to 120 °C. Roast the tomatoes for 30 minutes. Stir-fry paprika/bird-eye chili, garlic, red onion, carrot, and celery on 1 tsp olive oil. Once the vegetables have softened, add paprika and thyme. Add vegetable stock. Cook for another minute or two. Rinse your lentils and add to the pan until the mixture boils. Reduce the heat and simmer lightly for another 20 minutes. Stir regularly and add water if you feel like the mix is becoming too dry. Add kale to the mix, wait another 10 minutes, and stir in roasted tomatoes and parsley. Top with fresh arugula and drizzle with lemon juice and olive oil.

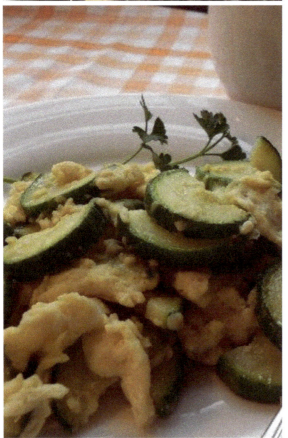

Eggs With Zucchini & ONIONS

Ingredients

- 4 eggs, Olive oil, 1 tsp
- 1 finely chopped onion
- 1 red chili pepper, finely chopped
- 1 finely chopped garlic clove
- 1 finely chopped zucchini
- Tomato sauce, 1 tbsp
- A pinch of salt, A pinch of Bird's eye chili powder and ground cumin
- Chopped tomatoes, 14 oz
- Canned quinoa, 14 oz
- Chopped parsley, ⅓ oz

Method

Fry onions and peppers up to five minutes in a thin layer of oil in a saucepan on low temperature. Add the zucchini and garlic, bring to a boil, and then add tomato sauce, salt, and spices. Stir and add quinoa and chopped tomatoes. Increase the heat to medium-high and let simmer for 30 minutes until the sauce reduces by a third. Remove from the stove, add chopped parsley, and preheat your oven to 200 °C. Add the eggs to the dish without stirring, cover with foil, and bake up to 15 minutes.

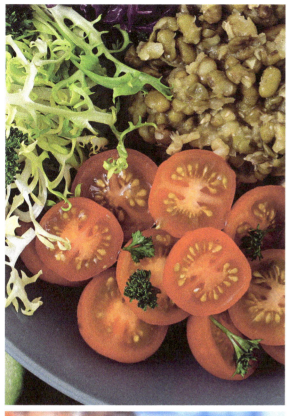

Tomato and Buckwheat SALAD

Ingredients

- Buckwheat noodles, 12 cup
- Arugula, 1 cup
- Basil leaves, 2 pieces
- 1 large chopped tomato
- Grilled tofu, 1 slice, chopped
- Olives, 12 cups
- Walnuts, ½ cup
- Extra virgin olive oil, 1 tbsp
- Lemon juice, 1 tbsp

Method

Cook buckwheat noodles per instructions on the packaging. Mix the remaining ingredients together to make a salad. Add drained buckwheat noodles and drizzle with the olive oil and the lemon juice.

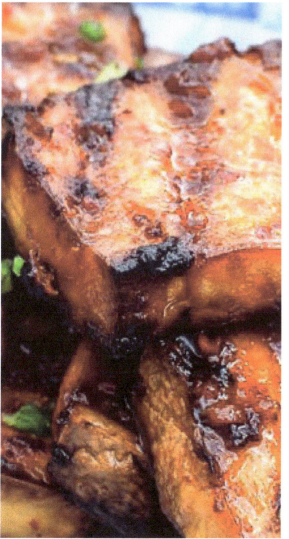

Grilled Mushroom and Tofu SUMMER SALAD

Ingredients

- Black olives, ½ cup
- 1 chopped tomato
- 1 chopped Bird's eye chili pepper
- Sliced red onion, ½
- 1 sliced cucumber
- Grilled tofu, cubed, 1 cup
- Mushrooms of your choosing, 2 cup
- Parsley, 1 tsp
- Basil, 1 tsp
- Ginger (optional), 1 tsp

Method

1. Grill mushrooms and tofu on a thin layer of olive oil for up to five minutes. Mushrooms can, but don't have to be fully fried, depending on the type.

2. Next, mix in the remaining vegetables and add the freshly fried mushrooms with tofu. Mix all together, add parsley, basil, and ginger, and drizzle with lemon juice and olive oil.

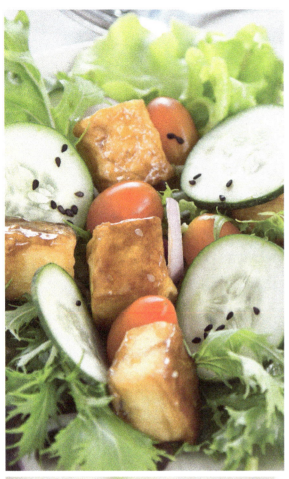

Sirtfood Tofu Sesame SALAD

Ingredients

- Sesame seeds, 1 tbsp
- 1 sliced cucumber
- Kale, chopped, 1 cup
- Arugula, 1 cup
- 1 fine sliced red onion
- Chopped parsley, ¼ cup
- Grilled tofu, diced, 2 cups
- Extra virgin olive oil, 2 tbsp
- Lime juice, 2 tbsp
- Soy sauce, 2 tbsp
- Raw honey, 1 tsp

Method

First, start by roasting sesame seeds for up to two minutes. Set aside to cool. If you've bought raw tofu, grill briefly on a thin layer of olive oil. Leave the remaining oil for salad dressing. Mix vegetables and spices into a bowl. Toss in the chopped grilled tofu and sesame seeds, and mix to distribute evenly throughout the salad. To finish off, drizzle with lime juice and olive oil.

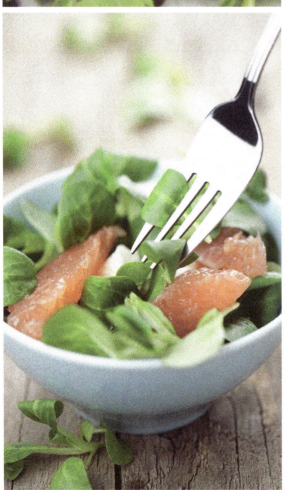

Sweet Arugula and Salmon SALAD

Ingredients

- Arugula, ½ cup
- Chicory leaves, ½ cup
- Lentils, 1 cup
- 1 sliced red onion
- Sliced avocado, 80 g
- Sliced celery, ½ cup
- Chopped walnuts, 1 tbsp
- 1 pitted, chopped, Medjool date
- Extra virgin olive oil, 1 tbsp
- Lime juice, 1 tbsp
- Chopped parsley, 1 tbsp
- Celery leaves, chopped, 1 tbsp

Method

Mix all ingredients into a bowl. Drizzle with lime juice and olive oil, spread on a large plate, and enjoy !

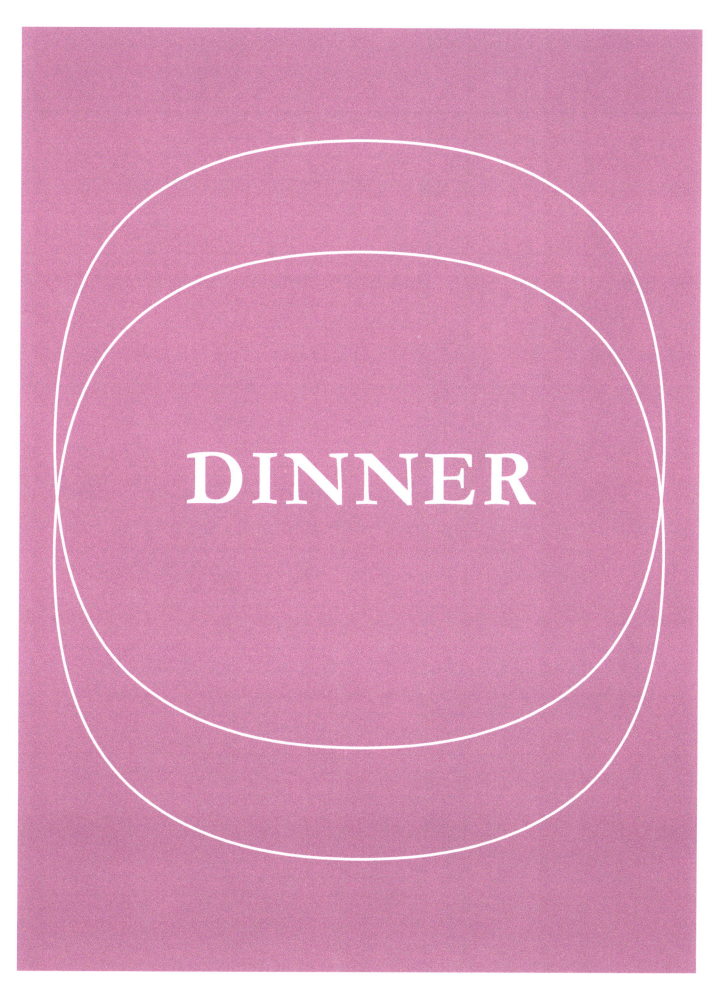

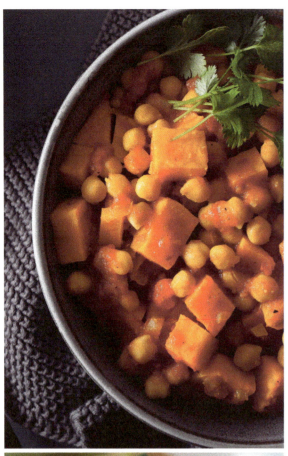

Sirtfood CURRY

Ingredients

- Skim milk
- Quinoa, 2 cup
- Chickpeas, 4 cup
- Potatoes, 14 oz
- Spinach, 1 ½ cup
- Tomato sauce, 1 tbsp
- 3 crushed garlic cloves
- Ground ginger, 1 tsp
- Ground turmeric, 3 tsp
- Ground coriander, 1 tsp
- Bird's eye chili powder, 1 tsp
- A pinch of salt
- A pinch of pepper

Method

Cook the potatoes for up to 30 minutes and drain. Move to a large pan and add all the ingredients except quinoa and bring to a boil. Once the mixture has boiled, add the quinoa and chickpeas, and up to 1 ½ cup of water if needed. Lower the heat and let simmer for 30 minutes while mixing regularly.

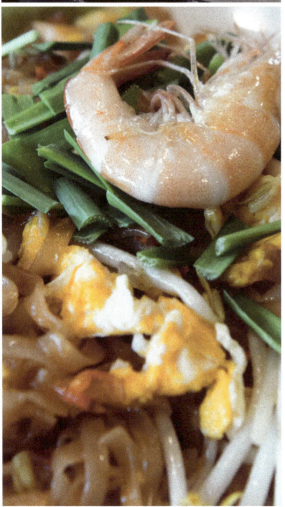

Buckwheat Noodles With TOMATO & SHRIMP

Ingredients

- Raw shrimps, 2 cup
- Buckwheat noodles, 1 cup
- Extra virgin olive oil, 1 tbsp
- One finely chopped garlic clove
- One finely chopped red onion
- Finely chopped celery, ¼ of a cup
- One finally chopped bird's eye chili
- Organic red wine, 2 tbsp
- Tomato sauce, 4 cup
- Chopped parsley, 1 tbsp

Method

Fry the garlic, onions, chili and celery in extra virgin olive oil for two minutes over medium heat. Add the red wine and tomato sauce and cook for another 30 minutes. Add water if needed. Prepare the buckwheat noodles while the sauce is cooking. Add pasta to the sauce when cooked. And the shrimps and cook for another four minutes. When the dish is cooked, add chopped parsley and serve.

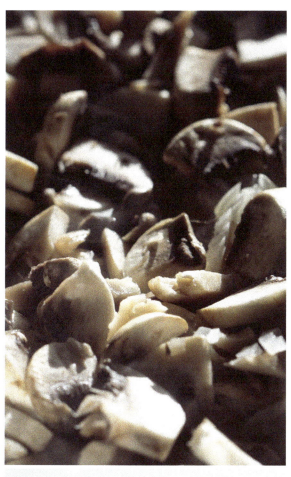

Onion Mushroom
SALSA

Ingredients

- Mushrooms, 1 1/2 cups
- Ground turmeric, 2 tsp
- Lime juice, 1 tbsp
- Chopped Kale, 1 cup
- 1 sliced red onion
- Arugula, 1 cup
- Fresh ginger, chopped, 1 tsp

Method

Fry the mushrooms on a thin layer of extra virgin olive oil for up to five minutes, while stirring and making sure they're cooking evenly. As you fry, sprinkle turmeric over the mushrooms. Add kale half-way through, letting it soften only lightly. Prepare a plate and lay out fresh arugula.

Mix the remaining ingredients together to make a salsa. If you'd like a more sauce-like consistency, you can blend the vegetables, spices, and the remaining oil. Serve one dish next to another and enjoy!

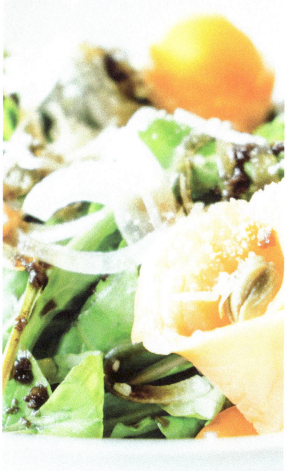

Arugula With
SMOKED SALMON

Ingredients

- Smoked salmon, sliced, 4 oz
- Chopped arugula, 1 cup
- Chopped parsley, 1 tsp
- 2 eggs
- Extra virgin olive oil

Method

Crack and mix the eggs. Roll slices of smoked salmon gently, and sprinkle with chopped parsley. Fry on one tablespoon of extra virgin olive oil briefly, up to two minutes on each side. Serve next to arugula and enjoy!

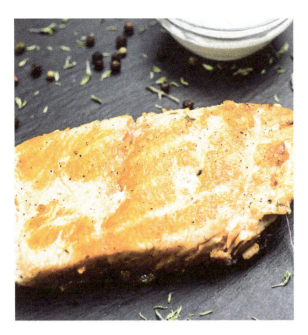

Sirtfood Striped BASS FILLET

Method

1. Rub the bass with olive oil and bake for 10 minutes at 220 °C.

2. Fry the remaining ingredients together (without say sauce and parsley) in a pan with remaining extra virgin olive oil. Once the green beans and kale have cooked through, add some water. Finish by adding soy sauce and parsley. Serve with the fish.

Ingredients

- Extra virgin olive oil, 2 tbsp
- Striped bass fillet, skinless, 7 oz
- 1 sliced red onion
- 1 finely chopped garlic clove
- 1 finely chopped red bell paprika
- Sliced celery, ½ cup
- Green beans, 1 cup
- Chopped kale, 1 cup
- Parsley, chopped, 1 tsp
- Soy sauce, 1 tbsp
- Ground turmeric, 1 tsp

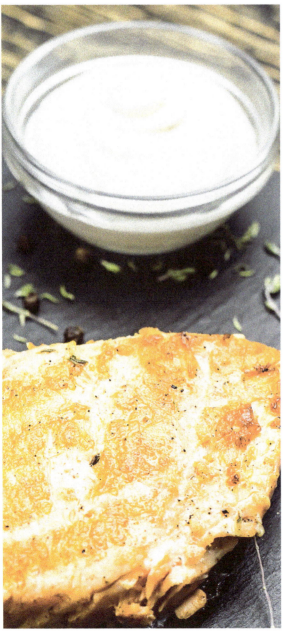

In this chapter, you learned how to eat Sirt Foods on a vegetarian diet. While the majority of ingredients for these meals are simple, easy, and affordable, it could happen that you can't find some of them in stores, or simply don't like a few of the original choices. For this reason, you can substitute ingredients as you like. The most important thing to keep in mind is that your meals should mainly consist of Sirtfoods. If you want to diversify your menu, you can use some of the recipes from the previous chapters. You can substitute meats for eggs, beans, and legumes of your choosing. Here are some general tips for making these recipes:

- *Stick to whole foods. Store-bought fruits and vegetables not only have less nutritional value, but also lack freshness, crunchiness, and consistency when cooked. It could happen that a pack of store-bought veggies has significantly less flavor than if you used organic options.*

- *Buy fresh foods. Frozen goods can contain a lot of water, and lose in volume once cooked. This can significantly impact the taste of your meals. If you're cooking with frozen foods, make sure to wait until they thaw, drain them to remove excess water, add more of the same ingredient if it has appeared to have lost some of its mass, and double-check the quantities before cooking.*

- *Be careful with fish and seafood. Food poisoning from fish and seafood is quite common, and equally unpleasant to experience. Always check the expiration dates on the packaging! The same can be said for making fish, shrimps, prawns, or clams. All of these, particularly if bought frozen, may lose some of their freshness once they thaw. For this reason, make sure to clean and drain the foods before cooking. If you're using frozen instead of fresh, you might find that the foods don't have as intense of a taste as you'd expect. This can happen with all frozen foods, and the best way to work around it is to add a bit more herbs and spices.*

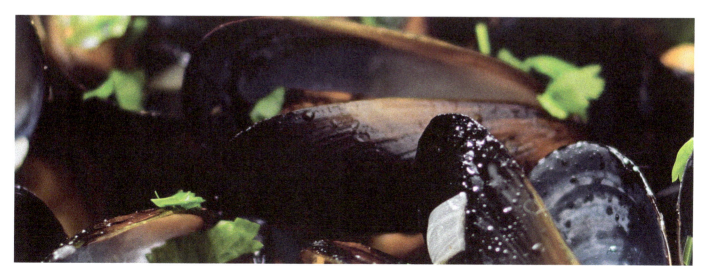

CHAPTER 5

VEGAN SIRTFOOD RECIPES

Don't eat animal-based foods? No problem! All of the known Sirtfoods are plant-based, and you'll have no trouble incorporating them into your daily diet. This chapter will feature Sirtfood recipes for vegans, but don't feel limited to these! You can use the recipes from the entire book if you substitute meat, eggs, and dairy with vegan alternatives. Without further ado, here are your Sirtfood meals from breakfast to dinner:

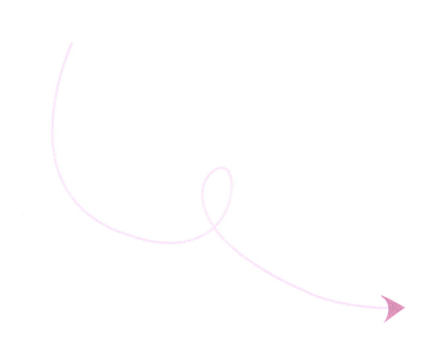

One of the common challenges of crafting a tasty, but calorie-dense breakfast, is to choose foods that are rich in healthy carbs and fiber, but don't have too much fat and sugar. In these recipes, we opted for buckwheat as the main source of carbohydrates, fruits to gain enough fiber, sugar, and vitamins (particularly strawberries), and different nut milks to alter the flavor of the smoothies the way you wish. Aside from adjusting other recipes given in this book, you can choose between these additional options on a vegan diet:

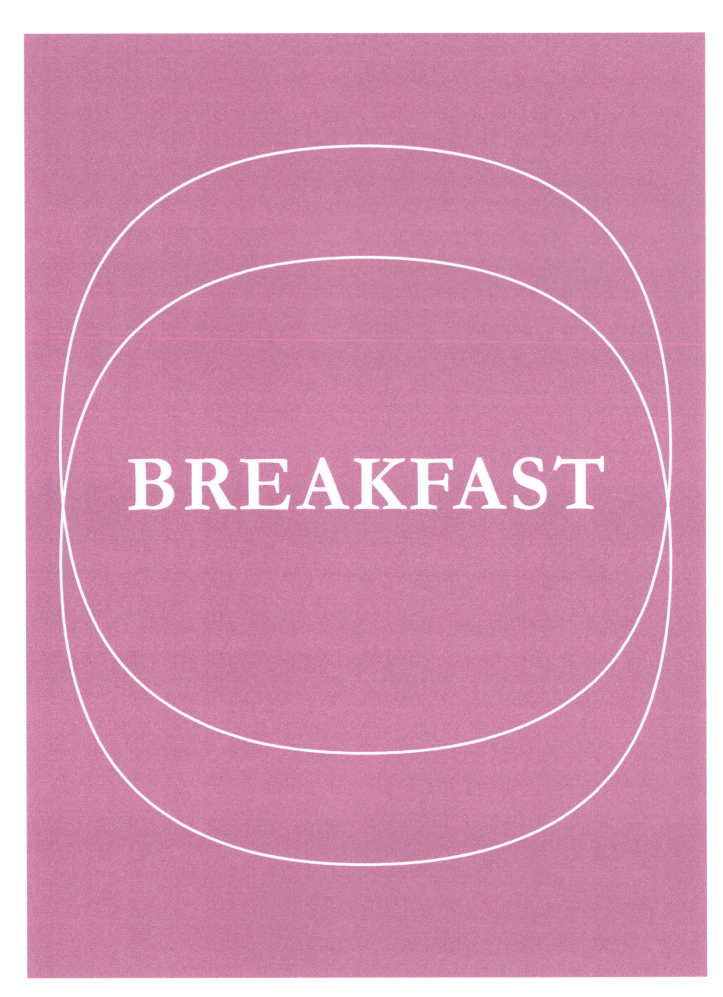

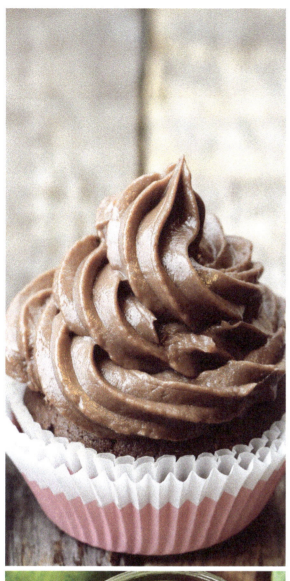

Walnut Chocolate CUPCAKES

Ingredients

- Buckwheat flour, 1 ½ cup
- Sugar, 2 cup
- Cocoa powder, 1 cup
- Salt, ½ tsp
- Almond milk, 1 ½ cup
- Vanilla extract, ½ tsp
- Coconut oil, ½ cup
- Walnuts, 2 tbsp
- Baking powder, 1 tsp

Method

1. Preheat your oven to 180 °C. Lay baking paper on the bottom of a cupcake pan.

2. Mix in flour, cocoa, and sugar and mix through. Mix in the vanilla extract, almond milk, coconut oil, walnuts, and baking powder and mix until the ingredients have combined into an even batter. Add boiling water and beat until it's evenly mixed in with the batter.

3. Your batter should now look quite liquidy, but don't worry!

4. Pour in the batter evenly across cake cases, filling up to ¾ of each case. Bake for up to 18 minutes and let cool.

5. Optionally, you can add vegan icing.

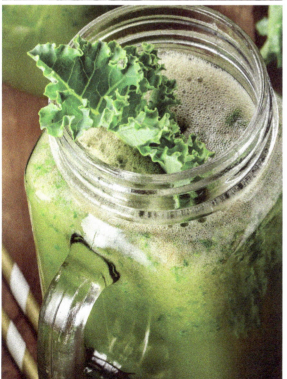

Sirtfood Kale SMOOTHIE

Ingredients

- Kale, finely chopped, 2 cup
- Raw honey, 2 tsp
- 1 banana
- 1 apple
- Fresh ginger, chopped, 1 tsp
- Half a glass of water, if needed

Method

Blend all the ingredients together and enjoy!

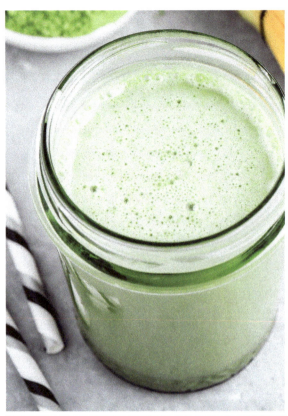

Fruity Matcha SMOOTHIE

Ingredients

- Matcha powder, 2 tsp
- Milk, 1 ½ cup
- Raw honey, 2 tsp
- Melon, chopped, two cups
- Mint leaves, fresh, 2-3 pieces
- Lemon or lime juice, 1-2 tbsp

Method

Pop all the ingredients into a blender, starting from the liquids to melon, and top with milk, spices, and lemon/lime juice. Blend all together and enjoy !

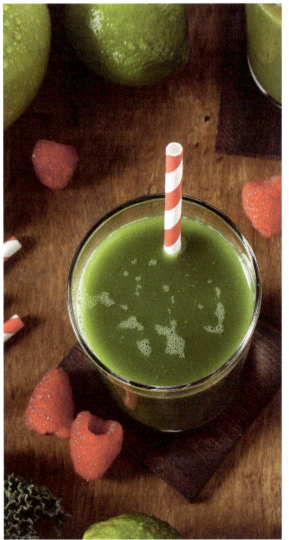

Fresh SirtFruit COMPOTE

Ingredients

- Green tea, fresh, ½ cup
- 1 lemon, halved
- 1 chopped apple
- Red grapes, seedless, 1 cup
- Strawberries, 2 cup
- Raw honey, 1 tsp

Method

1. Cook fresh green tea and 1 tsp of raw honey. Add the juice from ½ lemon and let cool.

2. Pour the grapes and strawberries into a bowl and pour the tea over the fruit. Serve after a couple of minutes.

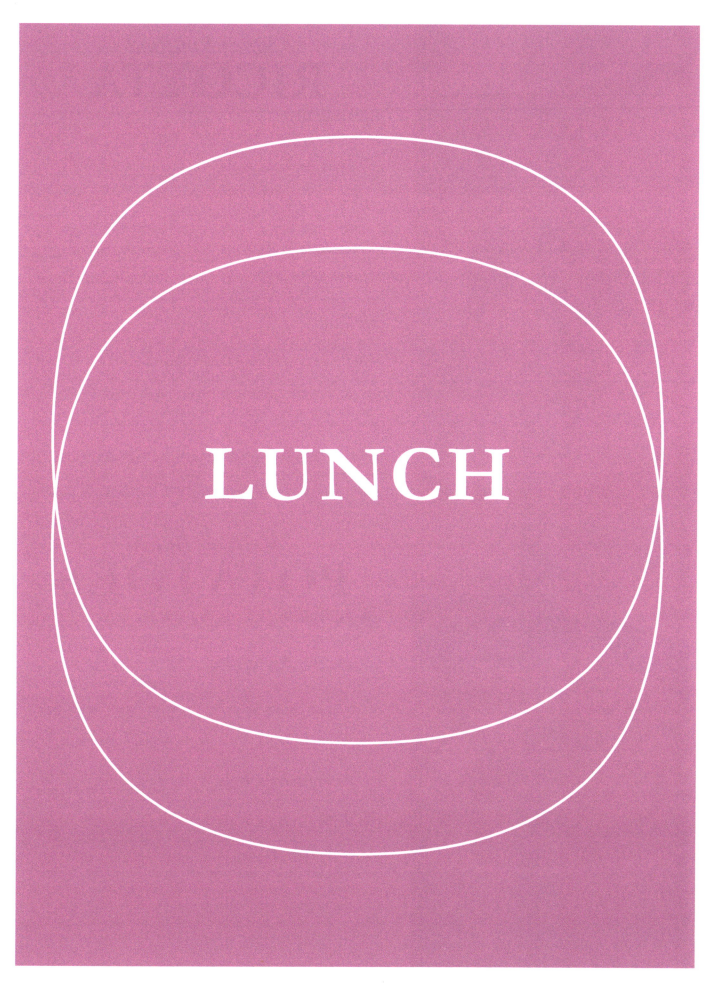

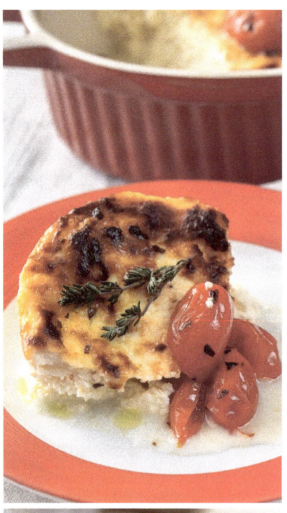

Spicy Sirtfood RICOTTA

Ingredients

- Extra virgin olive oil, 2 tsp
- Unsalted ricotta cheese, 200 g
- Pinch of salt
- Pinch of pepper
- 1 chopped red onion
- 1 tsp of fresh ginger
- 1 finely sliced garlic clove
- 1 finely sliced green chili
- 1 cup diced cherry tomatoes
- ½ tsp ground cumin
- ½ tsp ground coriander
- ½ tsp mild chili powder
- Chopped parsley, ½ cup
- Fresh spinach leaves, 2 cup

Method

1. Heat olive oil in a lidded pan over high heat. Toss in the ricotta cheese, seasoning it with pepper and sea salt. Fry until it turns golden and removes from the pan. Add the onion to the pan and reduce the heat. Fry the onion with chili, ginger, and garlic for around eight minutes and add the chopped tomatoes. Cover with the lid and cook for another five minutes.

2. Add the remaining spices and sea salt to the cheese, put the cheese back into the pan and stir, adding spinach, coriander, and parsley. Cover with the lid and cook for another two minutes.

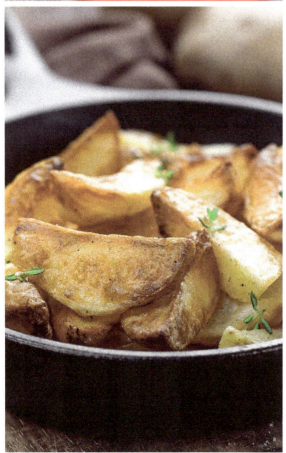

Sirtfood Baked POTATOES

Ingredients

- Potatoes, 5 pieces
- Extra virgin olive oil, 2 tbsp
- Organic red wine, 1 tbsp
- 2 finely chopped red onions
- 4 finely chopped garlic cloves
- Finely chopped ginger, 1 tsp
- 1 chopped Bird's eye chili pepper, Powdered cumin, 1 tbsp
- Ground turmeric, 1 tbsp
- Water, 1 tbsp, Tomatoes, 2 small cans
- Cocoa powder, 2 tbsp
- Parsley, 2 tbsp
- A pinch of salt and pepper

Method

Start by preheating your oven to 200 °C. Bake potatoes for one hour. In the meantime, fry onions in olive oil for five minutes until they're soft. Add chili, garlic, cumin, and ginger and cook for another minute on low heat. Add a tablespoon of water to prevent dryness. Mix in the tomato, chickpeas, pepper, and cocoa powder and let simmer for 45 minutes until the sauce becomes thick. Add parsley, salt, and pepper and serve with potatoes.

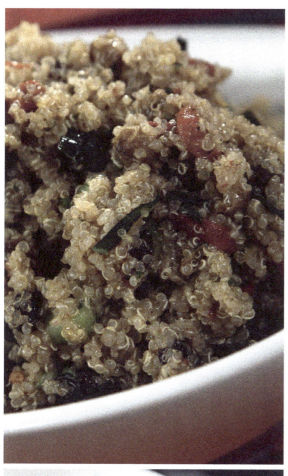

Spicy Quinoa With
KALE

Ingredients

- Canned quinoa, 1 can
- Extra virgin olive oil, 1 tbsp
- 1 sliced red onion
- 3 finely chopped garlic cloves
- 1 finely chopped bird's eye chili
- Turmeric, 2 tsp
- Coconut milk, 2 cup
- Water, 1 cup, Kale, chopped, 1 cup
- Buckwheat, 2 cup

Method

1. Fry the onions for five minutes in olive oil. Add ginger, garlic, and chili, and fry for another five minutes. Toss in the turmeric and wait for another minute. Then add in the quinoa and coconut milk, pour in a glass of water, and cook for 20 minutes. Add kale and cook for another five minutes.

2. Halfway through cooking the quinoa, fry the buckwheat in water for ten minutes. Drain and serve with the quinoa.

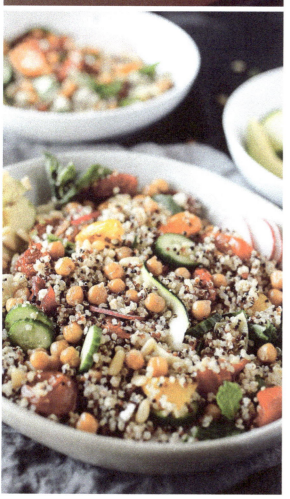

Mediterranean Sirtfood
QUINOA

Ingredients

- Quinoa, 2 cup
- Extra virgin olive oil, 1 tbsp
- Finely chopped garlic cloves, 1 tbsp
- Fresh ginger, chopped, 1 tsp
- 1 sliced bird's eye chili
- 1 sliced red bell pepper
- Ground turmeric, ½ tsp
- Ground cumin, 1 tsp
- A pinch of salt
- A pinch of pepper
- Chopped kale, 1 cup
- Lemon juice, 2 tbsp

Method

Start off by cooking the quinoa. Pour into a pot, cover with two parts water, and bring to a boil. Let it boil for up to thirty minutes. During the last five minutes, pan-fry the vegetables except kale in olive oil for up to five minutes. Once the vegetables have softened, add cumin, paprika, turmeric, salt, and pepper. Stir through and insert quinoa. Stir again, add vegetable stock, and pan-fry until the excess liquid vapors out. Serve and enjoy!

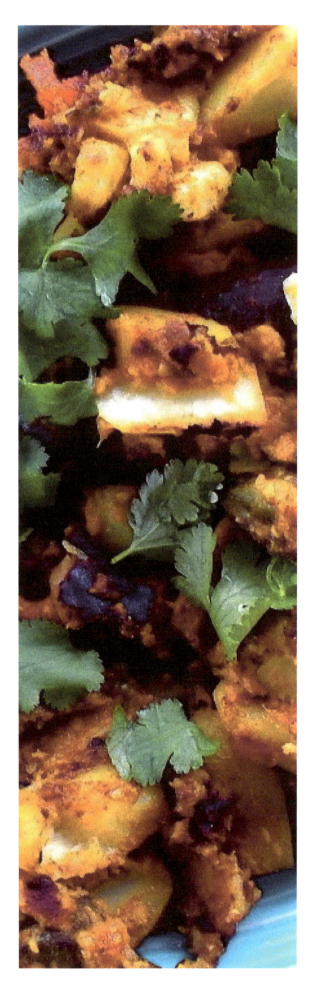

Eggplant and Potatoes in
RED WINE

Ingredients

- 1 large diced potato
- Finely chopped parsley, 2 tsp
- 1 sliced red onion
- Sliced kale, 1 cup
- 1 finely chopped garlic clove
- Sliced eggplant, 2 cup
- Vegetable stock, 1 ½ cup
- Tomato sauce, 1 tsp
- Extra virgin olive oil, 1 tbsp

Method

1. Preheat your oven to 220 °C.

2. Boil the potatoes for five minutes, drain, and roast in the oven for 45 minutes on 1 tsp of extra virgin olive oil. Turn potatoes over every ten minutes so that they cook evenly. Add chopped parsley once the potatoes are done.

3. Stir-fry the garlic, onions, and eggplant on olive oil for up to five minutes. Add the vegetable stock and tomato sauce, bring to a boil, and let simmer up to 15 minutes on low medium heat.

4. Serve with potatoes.

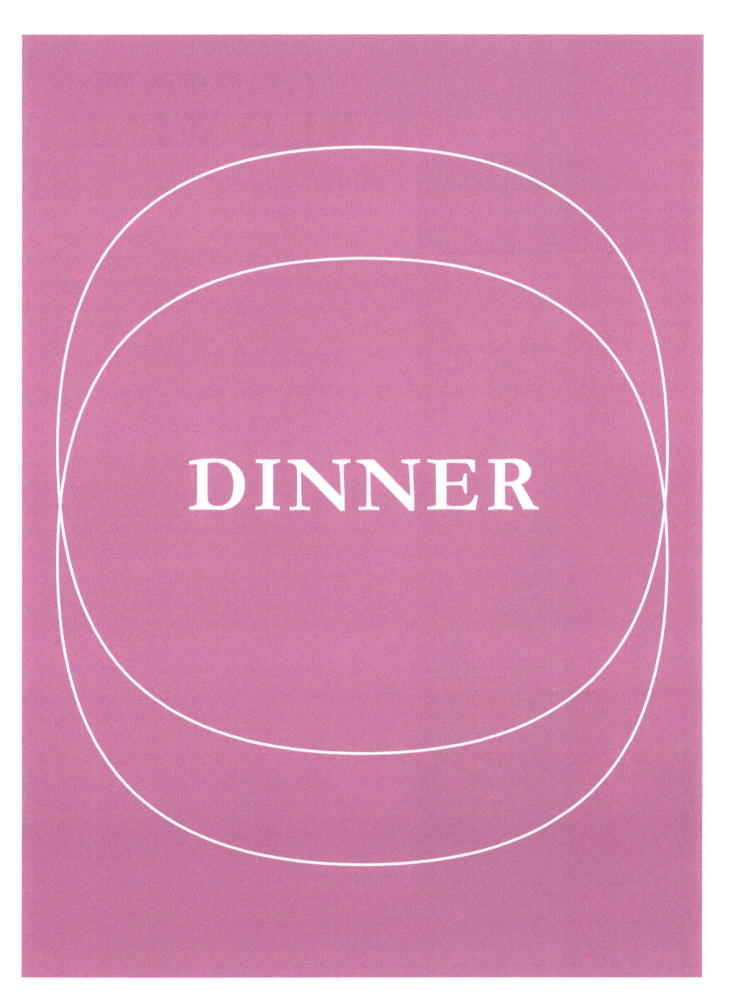

DINNER

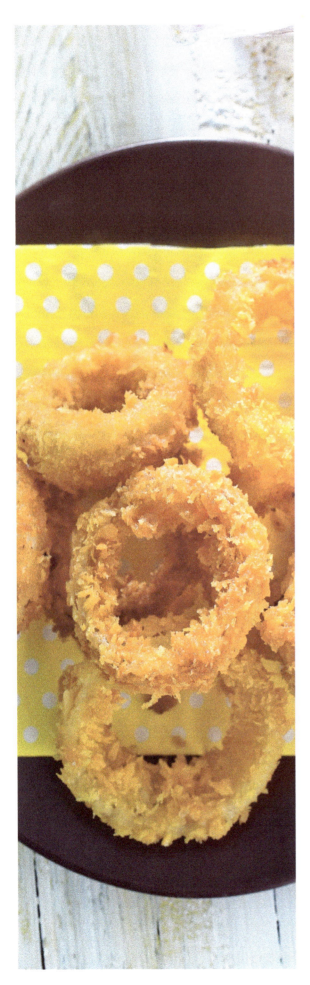

Potatoes With Onion Rings in
RED WINE

Ingredients

- Diced potatoes, 3 cup
- Extra virgin olive oil, 1 tbsp
- Finely chopped parsley, ½ tbsp
- Red wine, 1 tbsp
- Vegetable stock, 150ml
- Tomato sauce, 1 tsp
- 1 sliced red onion
- Kale, sliced, 1 cup
- A pinch of salt
- A pinch of pepper
- 1 chopped bird's eye chili

Method

1. Boil the potatoes for up to five minutes and drain. Roast at 220 °C for 45 minutes. Add the parsley after taking the potatoes out of the oven.

2. Fry the onions for up to seven minutes in 1 tsp of olive oil and add kale and garlic. Add vegetable stock and let boil for up to two minutes. Serve alongside potatoes.

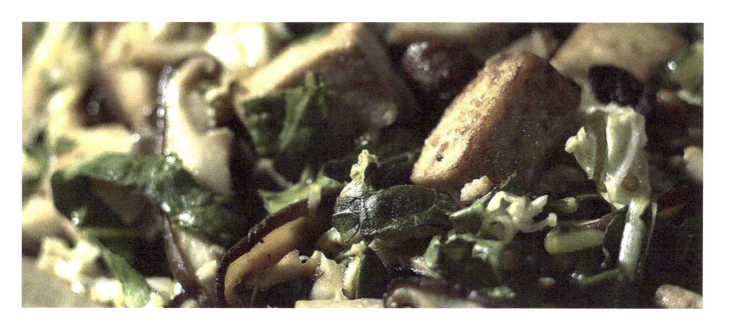

Sweet Potatoes With Grilled
TOFU AND MUSHROOMS

Method

1. Drain tofu by wrapping it in kitchen paper as you prepare other ingredients.

2. Cook buckwheat in vegetable stock. Add red wine, the tomato sauce, soy sauce, brown sugar, ginger, and garlic.

3. Stir-fry mushrooms for up to three minutes until cooked through. Add tofu and stir fry until the cheese turns golden. Remove from the pan and set aside.

4. Add the onions and stir fry for two minutes, upon which you'll add the diced sweet potatoes. Add more water or vegetable stock if needed, and add the sauce a minute or two before finishing. Combine the remaining ingredients and serve.

Ingredients

- Tofu, 14 oz
- Chicken stock, 1 cup
- Buckwheat flour, 1 tbsp
- Water, 1 tbsp
- Red wine, 1 tbsp
- Brown sugar, 1 tsp
- Tomato sauce, 1 tbsp
- Soy sauce, 1 tbsp
- 1 finely chopped garlic clove
- Ginger, finely chopped, 1 tsp
- Extra virgin olive oil, 1 tbsp
- Mushrooms, sliced, 1 cup
- 1 sliced red onion
- Kale, chopped, 2 cup
- Sweet potato, diced, 400 g
- Buckwheat, 1 cup
- Chopped parsley, 2 tbsp
- Vegetable stock, 2 cup

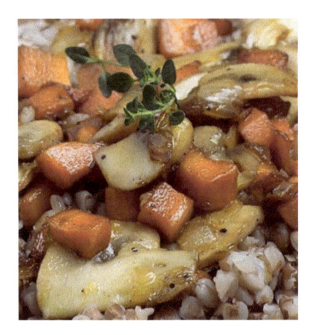

BUCKWHEAT STEW

Ingredients

- 1 finely chopped red onion
- 1 finely chopped large carrot
- 1 finely chopped garlic clove
- Finely chopped celery, 3 tbsp
- Extra virgin olive oil, 1 tbsp
- 1 finely chopped garlic clove
- 1 finely chopped bird's eye chili
- Vegetable stock, 2 cups
- Rosemary, ½ tsp
- Basil, ½ tsp
- Dill, ½ tsp
- Celery, finely chopped, 1 tbsp
- Canned tomatoes, 400 g
- Buckwheat, 2 cup
- Kale, chopped, ½ cup
- Parsley, chopped, 1 tbsp

Method

1. Fry the onions, garlic, chili, celery, carrot, and spice herbs in olive oil on low heat. Once the onion turns soft, add the vegetable stock and tomato sauce. Once the stock boils, add the buckwheat and let simmer for another half an hour. Add kale and parsley during the last five minutes.

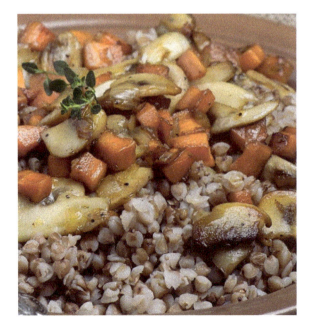

Cooking vegan on a Sirtfood regimen may look challenging at first, but the process can become easier and fun with some creativity. As with all other recipes, you're welcome to switch, substitute, and adjust ingredients per your own taste. Here are a couple of extra tips for more cooking inspiration:

- *Go for avocados. Avocados are very popular for those on a vegan diet because they supply plenty of natural fats and replenishing vitamins. But, for some, they're expensive or unavailable to buy on a regular basis. If this is your case, you can use bananas, melons, or sweet potatoes instead (depending on the recipe).*
- *Add nut butters. If some of the recipes given in this chapter are too lean for your taste, you can add nut butters or crushed nuts to the recipes. This will increase their flavor and add extra fat.*
- *Cook vegetables carefully . It might be tempting to let a dish simmer a couple minutes longer, but it's always better to steam or stir-fry as short as possible. Your vegetables are ready as soon as you can run a fork through them, and there's no reason to cook a second longer.*
- *Shuffle milks . You may get tired of coconut and almond milk. If you do, it's perfectly fine to use substitutes. Oat milk is one of the options you can go for as it won't significantly alter the flavor of the dish, but it will add sweetness. You can use soy milk as well, as it has a more neutral flavor.*
- *Explore mushrooms . Mushrooms are a great, lean source of protein, and you can choose from a long list of different species. They are easy and quick to prepare, and taste great overall. However, make sure to get mushrooms only from reliable brands and suppliers. They carry a risk from poisoning if grown near inedible mushrooms, and can cause great stomach discomfort past their expiry date. They are also heavily reliant on soil quality, which is why you should only buy organic ones. If you don't like mushrooms, you can always substitute them for artichokes.*

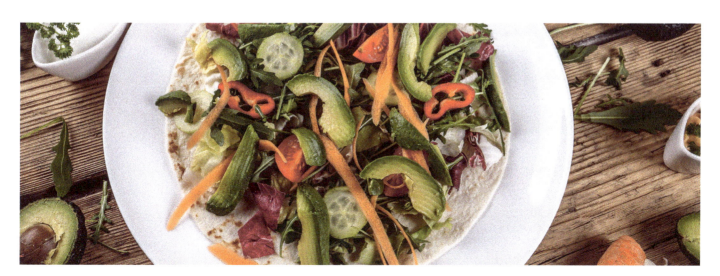

- *Spice it up! The recipes in this chapter feature a limited number of spices to ensure neutral flavors that will suit the majority of tastes. However, you can add any and all spices you like.*
- *Improvise with flaxseed. If you want to substitute animal-based ingredients from this cookbook, you can do so by mixing water and flaxseed meals in 3:1 ratio. This substitute will be great to substitute eggs so you can make your own vegan omelets and pancakes.*
- *Invest in organic foods. The Sirtfood program doesn't last forever, and since you'll be on a limited 1,000-1,500 calorie regimen, you won't use large quantities of foods, oils, and spices. Organic extra virgin olive oil, as expensive as it can get, is a great choice. You'll use it in almost all of your meals, and it's rich in nutrients and healthy fats. The same goes for coconut oil and herbs. Organic produce, while being more costly, is also richer in taste and smell, and it will secure a flavorful meal.*

*Now, **the best is saved for the very end**. The list of available vegan Sirtfood meals doesn't end with this chapter. In this chapter, you learned what to eat for breakfast, lunch, and dinner. But, what about those moments when you start craving sugar and sweets? This book's got you covered! In the last chapter of this book, you'll find recipes for delicious sweets and pancakes.*

CHAPTER 6

SIRTFOOD DESSERTS

It's one thing to eat clean and lean, but a completely different story to completely deprive yourself of sweets. The majority of diet plans fail because they don't acknowledge cravings for sweets. On most occasions, these cravings can be soothed by snacking on fruits, but not always. At times, you'll want to eat a delicious chocolate cake, or have some saucy pancakes. In this chapter, you'll find a couple of dessert recipes that are all based on Sirtfoods. These recipes are low-calorie, healthy, and easy to make. Enjoy !

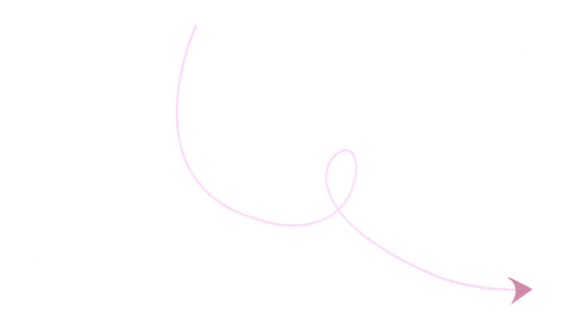

Sirtfood Walnut BALLS

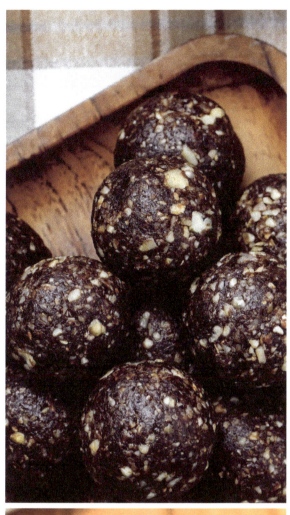

Ingredients

- Cocoa or almond milk, 1-2 tbsp
- Medjool dates, 2 cup
- Walnuts, 2 cup
- Vanilla, either one pod or 1 tsp extract
- Dark chocolate or cocoa nibs, 1 ½ cup
- Extra Virgin Olive Oil, 1 tbsp
- Turmeric, 1 tbsp
- Cocoa Powder, 1 tbsp

Method

Pop the chocolate and walnuts into your blender and process into a fine powder, adding milk and the remaining ingredients. Feel free to add more milk if the consistency of the mixture feels too thick, because this may depend on the freshness of the ingredients and individual package characteristics. Form the mixture into balls or any other shape and size of your choosing and roll in desiccated coconut and/or cocoa. This dessert can last up for a week in your fridge.

Sirtfood BROWNIES

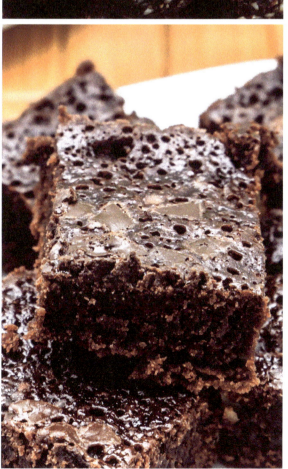

This delicious treat will take only five minutes to make! You will need to mix in a shortlist of ingredients.

Ingredients

- Walnuts, whole, 2 cup
- Almond milk, ½ tbsp
- Rum, 2 tsp
- Almonds, 1 cup
- Medjool dates, 2 ½ cup
- Vanilla extract, 1 tsp
- A pinch of sea salt
- Cacao powder, 1 cup

Method

Pour all ingredients together into a blender and blend until combined. Shape into balls, and either keep in your fridge for about two hours or keep in your freezer for around 30 minutes.

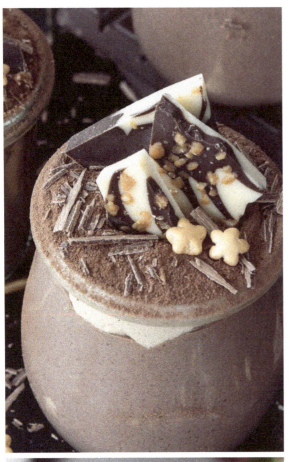

Sirtfood Chocolate MOUSSE

Ingredients

- Dark chocolate, 85%, 250 g
- 6 eggs
- Black coffee, strong, 4 tbsp
- Almond milk, 4 tbsp
- Chocolate flakes

Method

Place a bowl over a pan of simmering water. Melt the chocolate inside it, while paying attention not to touch the water with the bottom of the bowl. Remove the bowl and allow the chocolate to cool. Once the chocolate has cooled off, add egg yolks and the coffee and almond milk. Whisk with a mixer and add the egg whites gradually, while slowly mixing it with a spoon. Pour the mousse into glasses, flatten the surface, cover with thin foil, and cool for two hours. The mouse can also stay overnight. Sprinkle with chocolate flakes before serving

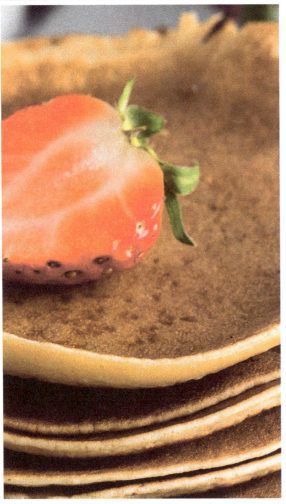

Chocolate Sauce and Strawberry PANCAKES

Ingredients

- Batter
- 1 egg
- Milk, 350 ml
- Buckwheat flour, 5 oz
- Extra virgin olive oil, 1 tbsp
- Dark chocolate, 85%, 3.5 oz
- Sauce
- Milk for chocolate sauce, 85 ml
- Double cream, 1 tbsp
- Extra virgin olive oil for the sauce, 1 tbsp
- Chopped walnuts, 1 cup
- Chopped strawberries, 4 cup

Method

1. Start by making the pancake batter. Mix in all the ingredients for the batter, pour into a blender and blend until smooth. You should have a batter of medium thickness, not too runny.

2. Start making the sauce. Place a bowl over a pan of simmering water, while making sure that the bottom of the bowl

doesn't touch the water. Place the chocolate in the bowl and melt over the steam. Once the chocolate has melted, add the milk and whisk for a minute. Add the olive oil and double cream.

3. Start making pancakes. Heat a frying pan until it starts to smoke. Insert extra virgin olive oil, and pour some batter into the center. Spread the batter across the surface of the pan. Cook for one minute on each side. Once the pancakes start lifting along the edges of the pan, use a spatula to lift and flip to the other side.

4. Once the pancakes are ready, spread the strawberries as you wish and roll the pancake. Layer the desired amount of sauce on top.

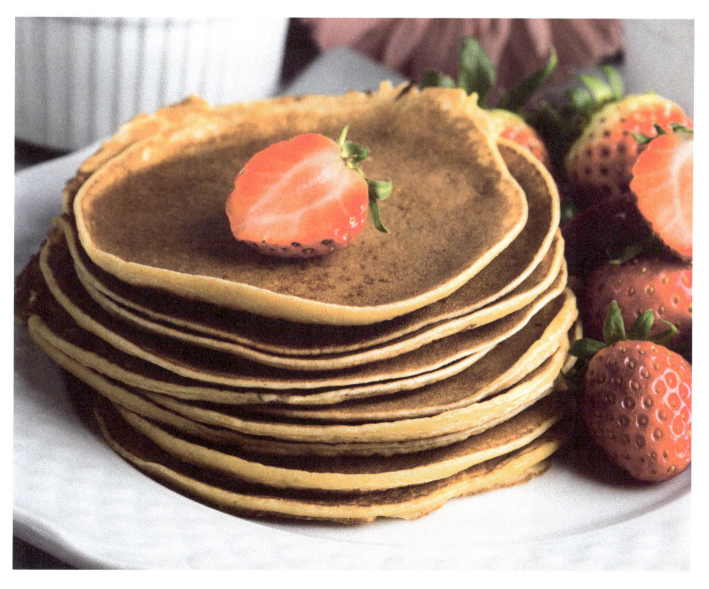

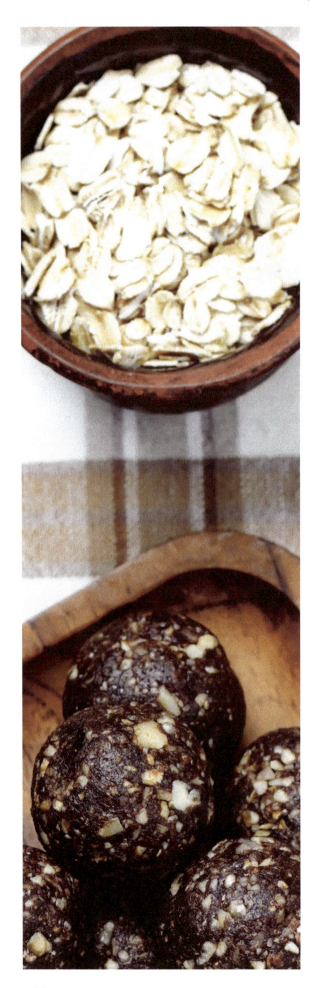

Cocoa and Medjool Dates
SNACKS

If you're one of those people who enjoy your afternoon sweets, these bite-sized cocoa balls will be a perfect substitute for your usual sweets.

Ingredients

- Dark chocolate, 70-85%, ½ cup
- Walnuts, 1 cup
- Pitted Medjool dates, 1 ½ cups
- Cocoa powder, 1 tbsp
- Vanilla extract, 1 tsp
- Water, 2 tbsp
- Extra virgin olive oil, 1 tbsp

TWO-WEEK MEAL PLAN
phase 1 and phase 2

Let's get to the heart and see a typical food pattern for the whole week. For each day, you will find indicated how much green juice to take and how to organize the main meals indicatively. As always, it is just an example to adapt according to your tastes and your caloric and nutritional needs.

phase 1

Day 1-3

- calorie intake is restricted to 1,000 calories.
- Three green juices per day plus one meal.

Day 1: Monday

green juice: 3 cups a day

- **Breakfast:** water + tea or espresso + a cup of green juice;
- **Lunch**: Green juice
- **Snack**: a square of dark chocolate;
- **Dinner:** Moroccan Chicken Casserole + vegetables and chicken.
- **After dinner:** a square of dark chocolate.

Day 2: Tuesday

green juice: 3 times a day

- **Breakfast:** water + tea or espresso + a cup of green juice
- **Lunch:** 2 green juices before dinner;
- **Snack:** a square of dark chocolate;
- **Dinner:** Sirtfood Bites + Coq Au Vin.
- **After Dinner :** a square of dark chocolate.

Day 3: Wednesday

green juice: 3 times a day

- **Breakfast:** water + tea or espresso + a cup of green juice
- **Lunch:** 2 green juices before dinner;
- **Snack:** a square of dark chocolate;
- **Dinner:** Salmon and Capers + chicken or fish;
- **After dinner:** a square of dark chocolate.

Day 4-7

- Calorie intake is increased to 1,500
- Two green juices per day and two more sirtfood-rich meals

Day 4: Thursday

green juice: 2 times a day

- **Breakfast:** water + tea or espresso + a cup of green juice
- **Lunch:** Sirt Muesli;
- **Snack:** a green juice before dinner;
- **Dinner:** vegetable soup with beans.

Day 5: Friday

green juice: 2 times a day

- **Breakfast:** water + tea or espresso + a cup of green juice
- **Lunch:** buckwheat salad with vegetables;
- **Snack:** a green juice before dinner;
- **Dinner:** grilled fish or meat + a side dish of vegetables and baked potatoes.

Day 6: Saturday

green juice: 2 times a day

- **Breakfast:** a bowl of that delicious Sirt Muesli + a cup of green juice
- **Lunch:** Sirtfood omelette with bacon;
- **Snack:** a cup of green juice;
- **Dinner:** chicken with walnuts and parsley + a red onion + tomato salad.

Day 7: Sunday

green juice: 2 times a day

- **Breakfast:** water + tea or espresso + a cup of green juice;
- **Lunch:** Sirt salad + grilled fish or chicken;
- **Snack:** a cup of green juice;
- **Dinner:** fish or meat cooked with a drizzle of red wine + plenty of salad and vegetables.

phase 2

- You should continue to steadily lose weight.
- No specific calorie limit for this phase.
- You can eat three meals full of sirtfoods and one green juice per day.

Day 8-15

- 1 x Sirtfood green juice
- 3 x main meals
- 1 to 2 light bites or appetizers and snacks
- 1 x glass red wine

Smoothie: Creamy Strawberry & Cherry Smoothie

Meal 1: Sirtfood Breakfast Scramble

Meal 2: Sirtfood Salmon Salad

Meal 3: Chicken Chili

Light Bites: Buckwheat Stir Fry with Kale, Peppers & Artichokes

Appetizers & Snacks: Avocado Deviled Eggs

Day 9-16

Smoothie: Mango, Celery & Ginger Smoothie

Meal 1: Sirtfood Breakfast Scramble

Meal 2: Sirtfood Salmon Salad

Meal 3: Chicken Chili

Light Bites: Buckwheat Stir Fry with Kale, Peppers & Artichokes

Appetizers & Snacks: Avocado Deviled Eggs

Day 10-17

- 1 x Sirtfood green juice
- 3 x main meals
- 1 to 2 light bites or appetizers and snacks
- 1 x glass red wine

Smoothie: Mango, Celery & Ginger Smoothie

Meal 1: Thai Red Curry

Meal 2: Chicken & Bean Casserole

Meal 3: Artichoke & Eggplant Rice

Light Bites: Apple-Nut Squares

Appetizers & Snacks: Creamy Peanut Dip

Day 11-18

- 1 x Sirtfood green juice
- 3 x main meals
- 1 to 2 light bites or appetizers and snacks
- 1 to 2 squares dark chocolate (85% cocoa)

Smoothie: Strawberry & Citrus Blend

Meal 1: Sirtfood Omelette

Meal 2: Chia, Quinoa & Avocado Salad

Meal 3: Foil Baked Salmon

Light Bites: Walnut and Onion Tartine

Appetizers & Snacks: Broccoli Cheddar Bites

Day 12-19

- 1 x Sirtfood green juice
- 3 x main meals
- 1 to 2 light bites or appetizers and snacks
- 1 x glass red wine

Smoothie: Mango, Celery & Ginger Smoothie

Meal 1: Honey Chili Squash

Meal 2: Brown Basmati Rice Pilaf

Meal 3: Mussels in Red Wine Sauce

Light Bites: Potato Rosettes

Appetizers & Snacks: Stuffed Dates

Day 13-20

- 1 x Sirtfood green juice
- 3 x main meals
- 1 to 2 light bites or appetizers and snacks
- 1 to 2 squares dark chocolate (85% cocoa)

Smoothie: Orange & Celery Crush

Meal 1: Cranberry & Orange Granola

Meal 2: Arugula, Egg, and Charred Asparagus Salad

Meal 3: Fried Sardines with Olives

Light Bites: Herb-Roasted Olives and Tomatoes

Desserts: Frozen Strawberry Yogurt

Day 14-21

- 1 x Sirtfood green juice
- 3 x main meals
- 1 to 2 light bites or appetizers and snacks
- 1 x glass red wine

Smoothie: Summer Berry Smoothie

Meal 1: Granola – The Sirt Way

Meal 2: Chilli Con Carne

Meal 3: Salmon and Capers

Light Bites: Walnut & Spiced Apple Tonic

Appetizers & Snacks: Tropical Chocolate Delight

Conclusion

Thank you for making it to the end. A healthy meal contains a lot of vegetables. So, most of the plate should consist of vegetables such as zucchini, cucumber, peppers or other vegetables, this guarantees a lot of vitamins, low calories, and a nice freshness (if the vegetables are not overcooked).

Colorful. Of course, it is not enough just to eat vegetables; it should also be varied and colorful. Ideally, the vegetables are as mixed and colorful as a traffic light: yellow, red, and green. Of course, a white vegetable such as white cabbage and cauliflower is not wrong and also serves as a colorful icing on the cake. The colorful mixture, which changes over and over again, also offers many vitamins and a varied taste. Even if you love something (such as tomatoes), it's important to vary a bit. Otherwise, deficiency symptoms can occur, and the food becomes boring over time.

Protein. Protein is one of the essential components of our body. However, not as much as needed, as many believe. And even then, it does not always have to be animal protein. Other sources of protein from beans and tofu provide a change in the daily diet and bring creativity to life.

Carbohydrates. Again, and again, the diets with "low-carb" (pronounced the "little-carbohydrates") the total hit. No wonder. Carbohydrates also make you fat. At least if you eat too many of them, if you eat them in the wrong combination (i.e., with too much fat or sugar) or do not vary enough. Carbohydrates are generally crucial in order for us to have energy, an essential ingredient for satiety, and it's important because it's good for your nerves, among other things. Of course

The best thing you can do for your body is to win food from natural ingredients. Fruits and vegetables are, at best, varieties that are available regionally and seasonally. Of course, it is okay from time to time sometimes not to eat regional specialties, such as pineapple or bananas (if you live in Germany, there will probably be hardly regional) but it is completely superfluous outside the strawberry time overpriced strawberries from Africa to buy, which taste like nothing and have hardly any vitamins.

As we end this book, please remember the five no-goes:

A lot of fat

Fat is good for the body. If we have too little fat, it will harm our health in the long run. But many people have the problem of eating too much fat which is not healthy either. Obesity is a modern disease that can easily turn into obesity. Too much fat is bad for the brain, the immune system, and the arteries, which in turn can cause a heart attack.

Of course, one must distinguish between healthy fats (olive oil, nut oil, nuts) and unhealthy fats (butter, animal fats, etc.). Because fat is not the same fat.

Lots of sugar

It is perfectly okay to consume sugar. Because sugar is an energy supplier, and sugar tastes good too. However, too much sugar is not good for the body, the immune system and can lead to addiction in particularly bad cases. Above all, sugar has the disadvantage that it does not fill you up for long and that you quickly lose energy again. Even if you are pushed by sugar, the effect lasts only very briefly.

Chemical substances

Our body is a natural organism; it does not need any chemical additives, so why should you forcefully pump yourself with chemistry? Unfortunately, for convenience, many people tend to stuff themselves with ready-made sauce-fix bags and other unhealthy things. From time to time, it may not be a problem to feed a little unhealthy; you will not die because you incorporate some e-substance. However, too many chemical foods are not good for your health. This can cause many other diseases of affluence that you would not normally have.

Many spices

People like spicy food, and that's perfectly fine, but certain levels of spiciness and too much salt are not among the spices people need on the contrary. The man needs a little salt. In fact, pretty much all foods contain some salt naturally and the over-flavoring of food causes water retention, is bad for the brain, and has a negative effect on the organism.

One-sided

The worst you can do to yourself, and your body is to eat one-sidedly. It does not matter whether the food bathes in fat, whether you are constantly fed on peppers, eating too much sugar or too little fruit, any form of one-sided diet has the result that you have deficiency symptoms, and you get sick sooner or later becomes. This can be in a one-sided diet, where you eat only unhealthy things and in a one-sided diet in which you eat only healthy food. Because one-sided is and remains one-sided. That cannot and should not be the goal because ironing out these deficiencies requires a lot of work and a lot of discipline.

That's all and I hope you have learned something!